Pregnancy Tales

Pregnancy Tales

Journeys into Parenthood

Edited by
Amy Tilston

Mercurist Publishing

Pregnancy Tales: Journeys into Parenthood
Copyright © Mercurist LLP, 2013
Copyright © Amy Tilston, 2013
Introduction © Tim Feest, 2013

Cover design by Amy Tilston and Tom Feest
© Amy Tilston and Tom Feest, 2013

All rights reserved.

First published in the United Kingdom
in 2013 by:
Mercurist Publishing
Hamble House
Meadrow
Godalming
GU7 3HJ
England

ISBN: 978-0-9926743-0-4

A catalogue record of the book is available
from the British Library

First edition: 2013

www.mercuristpublishing.com

Printed in England by Imprint Ltd, Seychelles
Farm, Upton Pyne,
Exeter EX5 5HY.

This book is dedicated to all the Mums and Dads who contributed their tales so freely and generously; and to their Mums and Dads, without whom...

...and to all expectant and newly-delivered Mums and Dads (and your babies!) in the hope that these tales will offer some reassurances, comfort and a modicum of practical advice for your own journeys into parenthood and childhood.

...and to our Little Dude, who arrived safely in the summer of 2012 and who delights and amazes us each and every day.

Contents

Foreword	vii
Acknowledgements	ix
Introduction	x
Note from the Editor	xi

Chapters

1	Meet the Mums	1
2	Getting pregnant	7
3	Finding out	11
4	Fran's Journey	15
5	Telling the world	46
6	First trimester	50
7	Advice	55
8	Mel's journey	58
9	Pregnancy symptoms	61
10	Plain sailing	64
11	Linsey's journey	67
12	Second trimester	73
13	What no-one told you about being pregnant	77
14	Kathy's journey	81
15	Sex, drugs and alcohol	90
16	Love it or loathe it?	95
17	Shellie's journey	99
18	Third trimester	117
19	Before and after	122
20	Thoughts about labour	127
21	Did your labour match your birth plan?	132
22	Labour painful	136
23	The unexpected	139
24	Top things to have for labour	143
25	Any other advice	146
26	If I did it again...	151
27	Birth stories	154
28	Meet the Dads	200

Some final thoughts and advice	209

Acronyms	211
Glossary of terms	213
Useful contacts	215
Index	214

Foreword

'What I wanted was a book that would tell me first-hand what other Mums and Dads went through; how they got pregnant; what it was like being pregnant; what labour was like; all of it.'

So said Amy, my oldest daughter, soon after she had given birth to her firstborn – and our first grandchild – in 2012: thus began our journey into print.

The Tales we offer here are almost entirely as they arrived from their authors. My role in its gestation (my, how using the terminology becomes automatic) has been to give advice on publishing and to act, willingly and gladly, as the sub-editor, tidying up the grammar and spelling and then formatting and typesetting the book for printing.

It has all brought back memories of starting our own family: that cold and frosty night in February when our first child, a son, was born after a rather short labour (we arrived at the maternity unit on Sunday evening at about 7pm and he was born some six hours later!). And then, thankfully for their Mum, a relatively short and not too complicated labour for each of the following three, of which Amy was Number Two...

Reading and editing the Tales has been an enlightening and, at times, a harrowing experience and I stand in admiration of all the Mums and Dads who have told us their stories.

It has also been uplifting and a delight to read how the new – and existing – parents coped with the various problems that occurred, particularly in labour (there always seem to be 'problems', big or small). I was pleased and not at all surprised to learn about apps for smartphones that can be used to monitor contractions; and as for TENS, well...you'll learn, if you don't already know what that's all about.

I was also quietly delighted to be reminded that giving birth is not a time for dignity and decorum: it seems that swearing and shouting, mostly at high volume, remains the norm for most Mums (and long may it continue); and it also seems that Birth Plans don't always unfold as expected. Our offspring, it appears, often still have their own ideas about how and when to arrive. Perhaps they start as they mean to continue...

Equally, I was amused and encouraged by the experiences of getting to the hospital – or not, if the staff didn't regard the Mum as being ready for admission. Amused, because it seems that often the understandable anxieties of new parents (I've been there!) were matched by the medical staff only when it was time to do so; and encouraged because when that time came, professional skills, knowledge and experience and the wonders of technology took over.

As a Dad, I salute those Dads who played their part, especially in labour and delivery. Back massages, high energy drinks (don't forget those bendy straws!), hand-holding and encouragement: all of this and more was evident, and rightly so.

To all of those who gave so freely of their time and their – often intimate – details, I add my thanks to those of Amy. I hope you will be as uplifted, reassured and perhaps moved to both smiles and tears as I have been in reading these Tales.

To all new Mums and Dads, I wish you every joy with your journeys.

Tim Feest
August 2013

Acknowledgements

My thanks are due to all the Mums and Dads who have contributed their stories: funny, sometimes heart-breaking and always truthful, they all tell a different pregnancy tale. Without them this book would certainly not have been possible.

To my Dad, who was the first to hear of my idea, and who has supported this project from start to finish.

To my husband for his patience, love and understanding. Our pregnancy journey was a steep learning curve for both of us but we got through it! He has become a wonderful father to our son and continues to support us both in every way possible.

Note from the Editor

All the pregnancy tales in this book have been submitted voluntarily by women and their partners who have experienced pregnancy and birth first-hand. Some names have been changed to protect identities but specific details have not been altered.

This is *not* a medical text book.

Medical conditions have, inevitably, been discussed, but if you have any concerns it is essential that you consult the relevant professionals and do not rely on the diagnosis of others.

The purpose of this book is to share with you our experiences and help you realise that each and every pregnancy and birth is different.

Amy Tilston
August 2013

Introduction

In the summer of 2011 my husband and I returned home from a long holiday in the Far East with a mission: Operation Baby #1.

Having thought about it before we went away, I was already taking my folic acid supplements and had begun to read up on the best foods to eat or avoid to maximise our chances. We hadn't thought much more beyond the positive pregnancy test, so when that arrived a mere two months later, it was suddenly a reality that our plan had worked!

A friend had recommended using the internet for extra support during pregnancy and I found that the two main sites in the UK were Netmums and BabyCentre. I plumped for the latter, for no particular reason, and began to trawl through the information and advice concerning pregnancy and babies. The most useful area soon became clear; the forums. I joined the 'July Birth Board' as this was when our bump was due and began reading and interacting with other parents due at the same time. From here I joined a group of like-minded women all experiencing pregnancy for the first time and all over the age of 30. Through this forum group we discussed our thoughts, fears, feelings and practicalities of becoming parents. Soon we realised that despite having come from different backgrounds, we all had a story to tell and experiences to share. Many of the stories in this book have been contributed by this group and I want to thank them for being my first source of inspiration.

It was from this group that I began to realise that what parents-to-be really want and need is reassurance. We are able to receive medical advice from doctors, midwives and health visitors but sometimes all we want to hear is that someone else has 'been there, done that' and has lived to tell the tale. I wanted women (and men) to be able to tell their stories; their 'pregnancy tales', in their own words without worrying whether what they experienced was medically expected or not. I wanted to give readers a chance to find comfort in the anxieties that we felt going through pregnancy and realise that sometimes being different is perfectly normal.

This book is therefore most definitely not a means of telling you what to feel or do at each stage of pregnancy and child-birth. It cannot mirror exactly how you are feeling, what aches and pains you do (or don't!) get or what it will feel like to carry a child for 9 months.

Pregnancy is a life-changing, exhausting, exhilarating and emotional journey. It will make you reassess your priorities, relationships and overall outlook of life. And this is all before your baby is born.

I believe our Pregnancy Tales are a truthful representation of what you could experience during pregnancy; but I'm sure you will find that your own experience is unique to you and your partner.

Amy Tilston
August 2013

Chapter 1

Meet the Mums

A brief introduction to the wonderful Mums who have shared their experiences throughout the book.

You can meet the Dads later!

Name: Louisa
Age (when pregnant): 33
How did you meet your partner? At work.
Did you always want children? Yes
ଔଔଔଔଔଔଔଔଔଔଔଔଔଔଔଔଔଔଔଔଔଔଔଔଔଔଔଔଔ
Name: Em
Age (when pregnant): 26
How did you meet your partner? At a bar in Manchester.
Did you always want children? Yes.
ଔଔଔଔଔଔଔଔଔଔଔଔଔଔଔଔଔଔଔଔଔଔଔଔଔଔଔଔଔ
Name: Jane
Age (when pregnant): 32
How did you meet your partner? We met in university in 2000. I saw him and thought 'he's alright' and that was it. We started dating shortly after and after 7 long years of waiting we got engaged in 2007. I had asked him before but he

was a traditionalist and didn't want me to propose. I wasn't bothered!!

Did you always want children? Yes

Name: Zoe

Age (when pregnant): 31

How did you meet your partner? In a pub.

Did you always want children? Yes.

Name: Jessica

Age (when pregnant): 30

How did you meet your partner? At a Lindy Hop dance class.

Did you always want children? I wasn't sure. I sort of fancied it but was always the one running away from other peoples' babies. And I had very good social life and wasn't sure if I wanted to give that up!

Name: Lindsay

Age (when pregnant): 36

How did you meet your partner? Through a friend at a festival, we had both broken up with partners recently.

Did you always want children? Yes.

Name: Lou

Age (when pregnant): 33

How did you meet your partner? At Sheffield University.

Did you always want children? Yes.

Name: Rachel

Age (when pregnant): 28 and 30

How did you meet your partner? Through church.

Did you always want children? Not especially

Name: Kate

Age (when pregnant): 36

How did you meet your partner? I was living in Paris at the time. We both went along to an event in a pub organised by a friend of friends and got talking and things went from there.

Did you always want children? I imagined myself with children without having a huge maternal instinct. Time went on and I kept myself busy with work, hobbies and far-flung holidays. As I got closer to 40 than 30 I thought that I should probably get on with things as there was a risk that I would miss out on something wonderful in my life.

Name: Natalie
Age (when pregnant): 30
How did you meet your partner? Online
Did you always want children? No

Name: Jenna
Age (when pregnant): 30
How did you meet your partner? On a dating website and then we met in a bar in Oxford.
Did you always want children? Yes, I felt ready and eager from age 16.

Name: Kathy
Age (when pregnant): 20–21
How did you meet your partner? We were on the same course at university. I'd been going out with another guy on the course for two years. We'd just broken up and Ollie asked me out for a date when he was drunk as a bit of a joke. He didn't think I'd say yes and was absolutely terrified on our first date.
Did you always want children? I hadn't thought much about it at the time – just assumed I would one day.

Name: Beth
Age (when pregnant): 33
How did you meet your partner? We were friends for a year before we got together. We had always liked each other but didn't want to ruin our friendship which is why it took a year.
Did you always want children? Yes.

Name: Emma
Age (when pregnant): 30

How did you meet your partner? At college when we were 16.

Did you always want children? Yes – although more so after I got married.

Name: Vicki

Age (when pregnant): 35

How did you meet your partner?
We were friends for about 13 years.

Did you always want children? Yes

Name: Laura

Age (when pregnant): 32

How did you meet your partner? Through a friend at work.

Did you always want children? Yes.

Name: Mel

Age (when pregnant): 35

How did you meet your partner?
He was my apprentice master at work.

Did you always want children? OMG no!

Name: Linsey

Age (when pregnant): 37

How did you meet your partner? In a bar, 5 months prior to getting pregnant.

Did you always want children? I always wanted kids and thought I'd missed the boat!

Name: Claire

Age (when pregnant): 26

How did you meet your partner? In the pub. It was ladies night, I told him I had a boyfriend as I'd just broken up with someone but then I got really drunk and announced to everyone how amazing it was to be single and he came over, Chablis in hand...

Did you always want children? Yes, always: I work with children and have always loved being with children.

Name: Cheryl

Age (when pregnant): 33

How did you meet your partner? On our way to a fete. We had a friend in common and at the last minute I hitched a ride with her to the fete. She stated that she had to meet some friends. He was one.

Did you always want children? Yes

ααααααααααααααααααααααα

Name: Liz

Age (when pregnant): 27

How did you meet your partner? Working at our local pub.

Did you always want children? Yes, I've always wanted two children (which I'm trying to convince Scott on, still!).

ααααααααααααααααααααααα

Name: Fran

Age (when pregnant): 30

How did you meet your partner? His sister and I worked at a local night club together and she had started to become friendly with my group of girlfriends. We all went out for said friend's birthday and she asked if her brother could come along. In he walked. A few hours and few drinks later I gave him 50p to ring his mother to tell her he wasn't coming home tonight (!).

Did you always want children? No, until I was 26/27 I was adamant I did not want them. I'm still unsure...

ααααααααααααααααααααααα

Name: Shellie

Age (when pregnant): 22 when first pregnant, 33 with second.

How did you meet your partner? I met my now husband and father of my second child in Ayia Napa on holiday when I was 19, we dated for a couple of months after but the distance was too much and he was 9 years older so felt at that point the age difference was too big, so we went our separate ways and lost touch.

We met up again on Facebook 10 years later! We had a drink to catch up as friends but it was like we had just met and fell head over heels all over again. He had moved nearer to where I lived, the age gap was not as apparent now I was older and after a year together, I introduced him to my first daughter who he adored as much as she adored him.

Did you always want children? Yes! I always knew I wanted to have children at some point in my life. I used to love playing with babies born in the family, loved babysitting every weekend as a teenager and totally adored my niece when my sister gave birth. However, unlike my parents who got married at 18 and had children at 21, I planned to get on with a career before settling down. My first child obviously was a bit of a shock so this didn't quite go to plan but I believe that everything happens for a reason and she really was the best thing that ever happened to me!

CBCBCBCBCBCBCBCBCBCBCBCBCBCBCBCBCBCBCBCBCBCB

Name: Christie

Age (when pregnant): 32

How did you meet your partner? Through DH's cousin who was a friend of mine.

Did you always want children? No. We'd said we probably didn't want kids at all then, when I was 30/31, I changed my mind. DH refused and we discussed splitting up (having been married for 7.5 years at that point.) I decided that I'd rather have him and no kids than the other way round so we stayed together. Then over the next year he gradually changed his mind. He says at first it was just to make me happy but by half way through the pregnancy he was more excited than me!

CBCBCBCBCBCBCBCBCBCBCBCBCBCBCBCBCBCBCBCBCBCB

Chapter 2

Getting pregnant

Starting a family is simple, right? Find yourself a suitable partner, have sex a couple of times and 40 weeks later out pops a baby....

Or not?

In some cases, yes, it can be that simple; we were one of the 'lucky' ones that took very little time (2 months) to get pregnant. For some, it was just as easy; for others, it took much, much longer.

The NHS advises that 84 out of every 100 women actively trying to get pregnant will be successful within a year. This figure increases to 92 in every 100 within 2 years and therefore anytime up to this point can be considered 'normal'. This doesn't take away from the heartache each month of a negative pregnancy test or an unwanted period. As you will see, some women took mere months to get their pink line, whereas some waited years and were either considering or had begun hormone treatment.

How long did it take you to get pregnant?

Six months
In the end, it took me a pretty normal time to get pregnant, but even so I did find it a bit disappointing and stressful when I got my period at the end of each month. After a number of months of no success I got a fertility monitor to know when the critical time was, and although it was not the most romantic way to go about things, it worked pretty quickly. (Kate)

5 Years
We had a missed miscarriage in 2009 which was discovered at 11 weeks. (Beth)

About **18 months**. (Louisa)

No time at all...We'd only been together a few weeks when I found out I was pregnant. [It was] completely unplanned and more than a bit scary! (Kathy)

We got pregnant **the first month** we tried. (Jessica)

About 2 years
I had been on Clomid to help me ovulate for four months and was having a month's break before starting IUI when we got pregnant. (Lou)

Just over a year
When I was 25 I was diagnosed with polycystic ovaries as I had not had a period since coming off the pill a year before. I was devastated as I was given no information from the doctors other than if I had not been successful getting pregnant within a year to come back.

After a few months of still no periods I did have two and thankfully the third never came as I was pregnant. (Em)

1 month (Natalie)

2 months (Laura)

3 months (Lindsay)

One year
We began trying in September 2010 and [I] fell pregnant in November but miscarried in February 2011. I fell pregnant again in September 2011 and we had a little girl in June 2012. (Vicki)

7 months
[We] accidentally fell pregnant before after being a bit lax with taking the pill but we were both happy. Unfortunately we lost that baby but at least it made us realise it was something we both really wanted. (Claire)

10 years
I was diagnosed with blocked tubes at age 25. I refused to have IVF for fear of being disappointed. Also, in my country [Trinidad & Tobago] it is not covered by insurance or a government plan. (Cheryl)

For this pregnancy: **three years**. I did get pregnant after 18 months of trying but unfortunately had an ectopic pregnancy resulting in the partial loss of my left tube.

This highlighted gynae problems so we were put on the IVF list and I had further surgery 6 months later to remove the rest of the left tube in preparation for IVF. Whilst in surgery they discovered I had endometriosis so the surgeon removed some areas of the endo and had to work to untether the remaining tube which was stuck down with adhesions.

I embarked on an alternative path to optimise fertility having regular acupuncture for stress, anxiety and fertility, took Agnus Castus herbs and followed a strict no-sugar diet as advised in the Zita

West Assisted Fertility book. The Agnus Castus was to help lengthen my luteal phase of my cycle which I had discovered was short through temperature charting my cycle.

2 months before IVF I fell pregnant naturally so as a result of the surgery and alternative things my dream had come true! (Jane)

Two months
We started trying for a baby in Sept 2009 and managed to get pregnant after two months – unfortunately I had a miscarriage at 7 weeks. We had a lousy Christmas in 2009 but we were positive about trying for a baby again as soon as we were able to. (Emma)

Three months
But every month it was a negative result was devastating enough! (Jenna)

Chapter 3

Finding out

Finding out for definite that you are pregnant can be a nerve-wracking business. According to our ladies the preferred method is to miss a period then 'pee on a stick'; but those few minutes of waiting for a line to appear or words to pop up can be torturous.

I had to wait for my husband to return home from a work trip in the States. Like others I was waiting for my period to come but I had a sneaky feeling that we had been successful this month. I wanted to use a digital test as having the words 'pregnant 3+ weeks' appear was just fantastic.

How did you find out you were pregnant?

I began to suspect that I was pregnant when I kept feeling like I was about to get my period but nothing happened. I kept my thoughts to myself for a few days, as I didn't want to tempt fate. We were away for the weekend at a cheese festival and on the Saturday morning I said to my boyfriend, 'I think I might be pregnant'. I had a pregnancy test at home, so had decided that I would use it on our return. In the meanwhile, the cheese festival proved a bit complicated, as I knew that there were certain cheeses that I couldn't eat, but I wasn't sure which ones. When we got home, I immediately did the test, and it very quickly came up with 'pregnant'. (Kate)

I bought a bag of dip sticks and started testing 6 days before my period was due. I got a very faint line that day then a stronger line the next day then bought some proper tests and did those in the evening to confirm. I showed my husband first then ran to ring my sister and best friend! (Christie)

I was counting down the time on a flight home from an all-inclusive holiday in Cyprus, and then did a pregnancy test as soon as I got into my house. (Natalie)

I was at home, Stuart was in Milan on a work trip, I sent him a picture of my pregnancy test but he couldn't figure out what it was! (Claire)

I was a week late so did a test thinking there's no way I was pregnant after such a short amount of time and bingo, I was!! He didn't believe me at first! Then as I had peed on the results window and the lines were faint, the instructions said this could affect the result, so neither of us knew if I was actually pregnant until the next morning when I went to Boots near to work to buy another test. I really panicked that someone from work would see me! I then had to do the test in the work toilets and yay, it was a Big Fat Pregnant!! I emailed my husband as obviously I couldn't call him from my work phone and he was over the moon, we both were! (Lindsay)

I was doing pregnancy tests all the time and eventually one was positive! I was at home but my husband was out all day so even when we spoke on the phone I had to wait until he got home to tell him. (Laura)

It was 6am in the bathroom on Halloween. I'd decided to do a test as I was a few days late (unusual) and was due to start fertility treatment that Friday. I thought it was best to do a test so that I wouldn't be wasting the clinic's time. (Beth)

I found out I was pregnant after having a drink with a friend when I got home. I had previously taken a test the week before but it had shown it was negative. I took the test [again] because my breasts felt sore when I went for a run. (Em)

I had sore boobs and did a pregnancy test. (Louisa)

I was on holiday with friends in Majorca in October 2011 when I missed a period. (Vicki)

I missed a period so called into a chemist to pick up a pregnancy test 'just in case'. I hadn't done one before and didn't really think I was pregnant but wanted to be sure.

It was a bargain-basement kit they had on offer – really basic – and I did the test in a public toilet on my way to work in the evening.

The marker was meant to take a few minutes to develop but the line came through very strongly immediately. I was quite distracted at work that evening. (Kathy)

In a Tesco toilet off the M25 on the way home from teaching on a course – classy! (Jessica)

We had been trying to get pregnant again for a couple of months and I had an inkling we had been successful – we went into Manchester to watch Peter Kay at the MEN and had gone through early to get something to eat. We decided to get a pregnancy test and decided we couldn't wait until we got home to try it. I went to the bathroom and took a positive test, we were both really pleased. (Emma)

[My] period was due on Tuesday 25th October. During sexual relations on the 24th I started bleeding. On Friday 28th while sitting at my desk I got ill when I smelled a chicken sandwich being microwaved. I ran and threw up and realised that my period had not come after all except for the spotting. After work I bought a pregnancy test which I took at midnight and got a BFP... Yay! (Cheryl)

I had felt a lot of pain the two days before I tested and thought it was my period. When that didn't arrive I woke on the Sunday morning and felt I wanted to go to mass so I went and lit a candle and said a few prayers. On the way home I picked up a test in Asda and said to my DH I have a feeling. I took the test and there was a faint positive. I was thrilled but very nervous as I knew another ectopic would have to be ruled out first. (Jane)

One morning doing a test at home with Ben, very undignified, both half dressed, with me on the loo. (Jenna)

Chapter 4

Fran's journey

Because it is estimated that around one in six couples in the UK (approximately 3.5 million people) will have difficulty conceiving naturally, I wanted to include the story of a couple's journey through assisted conception.

The following journal has been taken from an online diary and chronicles the emotional stages encountered in one couple's attempts at becoming parents. It begins three years into their journey. As with all the pregnancy stories in this book, this is a personal and unique experience. If you feel you need help conceiving then please see a doctor to discuss your options.

For the purpose of authenticity the acronyms and abbreviations used have been left unaltered: there is a glossary of terms at the end of the book.

13th September 2009
Only Two for Christmas This Year

When we were little, we used to have Easter egg hunts round the garden on Easter Sunday and we used to have to find them after my Dad was hiding them. Then the five of us would sit down around the table and make sure that we all had our fair share of eggys then we'd sit eating them watching cartoons 'til Mum cooked dinner.

Yesterday it dawned on me that I won't have kids to do this with for at least another two Easters, by the time they're born and old enough for an egg hunt.

Made me feel a little sad, because what follows that are thoughts of two of us round the Xmas dinner table AGAIN this year!! Every year when I put the Xmas decs away up in the attic, I write myself a letter. It says what has happened this year, what I hope will happen in the coming year. It's nice, like a little time capsule. And for the past three letters I know I have written:

'Maybe this will be the last year there's only two of us.'

26th September 2009
Cycle 33

Just feel like I need to write this month down. I'm trying not to symptom spot but after having my 1st ever +ve OPK on CD15 this cycle I feel the need to indulge myself a little to keep my PMA going.

I'm hoping this is my month as I'm still waiting for a referral to the fertility clinic from my local hospital and secretly hoping I won't need it.

CD10 – 1st ever Reflexologist session.

CD14 – BD at night.

CD15 – Peak and very strong +ve on OPK

CD16 – BD – 2nd peak OPK faded from yesterday.

CD17/1dpo – full, bloated feel in lower belly, slight cramping and niggly feeling.

CD18/2dpo – cramping feeling in my belly, and slight lower backache, coupled with being a moody cow and sneezing. Feel as though AF could be starting but know that's impossible, also felt pop feeling and just feels like there's something going on down there iykwim.

CD19/3dpo – still feeling like AF type cramping and back, dull ache in left side but this happens every month. No CM, feel like it's there but it's not – PMA drifting away!

CD20–23 – On hols, no SS.

CD24/8dpo – Have felt like AF is coming, back and front, when I was at the loo earlier I wiped and it was tinged pink, gutted she's coming and 3 days early.

CD26/10dpo – Small pink bleed at 8am-ish, couple during the morning but nowt in afternoon, I suspect full flow by 2moro morning, boobs are sore and heavy as usual. Small light red bleed in evening.

CD27/11dpo – Same light occasional bleeds on and off through the day. Nothing like strong constant flow of an AF, no dark stuff, no constant flow. I did have occasional AF type cramping and backache which made me think the witch would be here. Also loose bowels.

CD28/12dpo – Light bleeding went to spotting mixed with brown stringy type of EWCM stuff! Loose bowels again.

CD29/13dpo – No bleeding from 5pm yesterday 'til 9am this morning (7/10/09) when I had some red when I wiped. Starting to think I'm being stupid and I need to accept that it was just a really light AF but the fact my boobies are still hurting is making me think otherwise 'cos they normally stop when she comes.

BFN with eBay cheapies with FMU.

13th December 2009
A Realisation or Two...

With January approaching, it will mark our 3 years of TTC.

Wow, 3 years...

For the past few Christmases I have wondered if this will be the last one with just the two of us. But it dawned on me literally half an hour ago that during these 3 years I have not had an MC or a chemical (to my knowledge) and can only therefore assume that there is something seriously amiss with us.
So, with fertility testing well underway, there is a glimmer of hope at the back of my mind that even if we have to pursue the ICSI/IVF route, surely it can't take longer than a year?
So I find myself whispering back to myself,

'Maybe this will be the last Christmas there's just the two of us?'

This time next year I will be busy buying baby clothes and apparel and decorating the baby's room and sporting a bump or be nursing a newborn.

How long will it take 'til this glimmer of hope fades?

We have everything to give to our baby, a loving family and nice home, earn enough money to make sure that he/she doesn't go without.

I can laugh it off and brush off the day to day feelings of emptiness that I feel every time I see an unexpected bump pass by, or next time I gaze into the big empty spare room at the back of the house that is desperate to have a young Sull in there?

Is this it? IS this the last empty Christmas? The last Christmas there's just us two?

We'll see.

31st December 2009
Cancelled Christmas 2010

I've taken my tree down on New Year's Eve and decided that Xmas is for kids and if I don't have any or am not PG by next Xmas then there will be no tree, dinner or presents under my roof next year! Balls to you, Santa!

I've got to take a stand for my sanity as in 3.5 hours (Jan 2010) I would have been TTC 3 FEKKING YEARS! I am sat here on yet another CD28 waiting for the effin' bitch to show up, NO MORE I yell!

I have had enough of this waiting shit!

Bring me my baby NOW!

NOW, I TELL YOU NOW!!

Yes, I've been a little bonkers this past week and it's been added to since I found out that the nearest private fertility clinic treatment is about £4k!

God damn it, I've waited enough now! At least no one in the immediate family had announced they're PG. I'm waiting for DH's older sister to announce it and I will then become an alcoholic!

And breathe.

Happy Effin' New Year – Bah! Humbug!

24th January 2010
Is It Time To Stop?

Has the time to come to stop TTC?

I have been talking to a friend tonight and think that my end is near. I'm wishing my life away cycle after cycle, waiting for 2 lines to appear, not paying attention to everything else life has to offer.

Yes, it could be possible I'm on a down day, but I really think that depending on what the FS says on 23rd Feb I will be calling it a day, but I know the only way I can really do that is by leaving BC, getting a clean slate and leaving everything behind me.

I felt like this knowing my 3 year mark was approaching but now it's been and gone I believe it's all a reality check and I need to accept things and move on, there's only one life we've got and I'm wasting mine away wondering on the ifs/maybes/whens and I think it's enough now.

This cycle coming up could be the last one I share with my BC community, the beginning of the end.

23rd February 2010
The Next Step

Finally had my 1st appointment with my actual consultant and I needn't be concerned, she was nice enough, it had only been postponed a month but felt like a lifetime.

She said that there's nothing in all the results so far that would stop us being PG which is great, she wants to do the lap and dye next. She will be checking for Endo (endometriosis) and giving the tubes a bit of a flush, and she said that there's about a 60–70% chance of getting PG afterwards which I knew but was nice to hear from a pro.

Unfortunately there's a 3–4 month waiting list, but what's another few months right? And they have my mobile number so if they get a cancellation it could be sooner. It'll be in the day surgery unit and I will be knocked out (eekkk!) but if that's what's got to be done next then so be it.

I bought myself some Pregnacare Conception for this cycle so I will stick to that and haven't had any mid cycle spotting this month which is good.

Had a rough few weeks so it's a good bit of progression I think. Now it's moving on there's nothing more I can do so let's just roll with it.

7th May 2010
Why is this Journey such a Rollercoaster?

I feel schizophrenic!

That's the only way I can really describe this!

Holy hell!

One minute I want to pack up my BC account, go buy some Durex and forget all about this TTC malarkey – and then on the next breath I am at OV time, EWCM galore and walking around with a smile on my face because I'm wondering if this will be my month?!

How can I still wonder if this will be my month after 40 MONTHS!

This is cycle 40!

Jeez – and then I wonder why I find it hard to keep my PMA and I feel bad for feeling a bit off every few months?! PAH!

C'mon mun – Where's our baby?!

24th May 2010
Next Step: Lap & Dye

So after what I feel has been a REALLY long wait, I am CD4 today and going in for my lap & dye Weds morning.

I'm not nervous, I actually feel slightly excited. I 'feel' deep down that this is what we need.

Imagine: I've been having sex with DH for 10 years, all that stuff blocking up and messing up my tubes, I hope the dye will give them a good flushing.

Do you think I can ask the FS to take some pipe cleaners in with her to give them a scrubbing while she's there?

I think I will give myself this month off to repair and relax and jump back on with the next cycle.

It's actually quite invasive when you think about it, pumping my belly full off gas to get in there and have a look. I wonder if they'll laugh and point at my naked body whilst I'm under.

So here's to joining the March 2011 BB.

27th May 2010
Lap & Dye: What Happened and Results

I forewarn you now, this will be detailed and as thorough as I can make it, so other girls can relate and I can remember.

I had to be at the day surgery unit by 8am. When I got there I was booked in, gave them my sample of FMU to test with, had my BP taken and then waited.

8.15am: Met with registrar who went through consent form and explained to me what they'll be doing and why, then straight into anaesthetist for pretty much the same. Told I was second to go in. Both nice enough guys, I felt totally chilled.

9.15am: Am told to change into the sexy theatre gown and my dressing gown, stripped off, popped it on along with a lovely pair of theatre socks lol. Sat back in waiting area, really could do with a drink and brekkie at this point but no chance.

10am: I am called for the long walk down to theatre. I was told that a standard lap and dye test can last about 20 minutes, if anything's found then I won't be in there longer than an hour. I walked into theatre to be met by the anaesthetist and his dude and they were both lovely. Strapped me down, stuck a drip in my hand, was told they're putting stuff into me now that'll make me drowsy, I remember everything going fuzzy and I was outters! Very cool.

11am: I remember coming round and starting to cough 'cos of the tube down my throat, I don't think they expected me to come round so quickly. So I had a nurse by the side of me for the next 15mins to make sure I was ok, testing my BP, etc, and then she said 'So they got all your Endo then', I was like HUH?! Did they find some then? My throat was so, so sore and dry beyond belief so I didn't really understand what she was saying.

11.20am: Laid in recovery pleading for water and having my BP checked. Asked for my handbag so I could let DH know I'd come out ok. My head was still spinning at the thought of Endo?!!?

12pm: Registrar started to come to see the 3 of us gynae patients. Listening to next door, she had the all clear. Then he came to me.

> 'Everything went fine', he said, 'but we did
> find some endometriosis.'

I was a bit shocked to say the least. He said it was around both ovaries, a few spots scattered around and also covering the ligament to the uterus. He then showed me pics of it all (haha!). He said he'd lasered it all away. I will now have to go see my FS for a more in-depth explanation I expect. Don't know how long that's gonna be. He left.

12:30pm: Text everyone to say I was awake, DH text I love you and I started crying. OMG, is this the reason we don't have babies? Has this been hindering me all along?
Feeling very emotional.

1:30pm: I eat a VERY dry cheese sandwich and ask to get up and dressed. This I did and then I sat in the waiting room 'til 6pm and waited for DH to pick me up. At 4pm I was sick lol.

By the time I got home, had some toast and took my drugs I went to bed, I had nothing in me and needed to rest.

My first reaction was joy at having a problem found and fixed, but now as I read and research, I don't think I will get PG naturally.

Hope it's not too long 'til my next appointment.

28th May 2010
2 Days Post Lap & Dye – Feelings and Thoughts

Just thought I would add to my entry and explain how I feel two days later.

Physically I'm good, I have four lots of stiches in three areas, all of which we cleaned and re-dressed yesterday. I wanted to look just so I know what I'm dealing with. I have had slight twinges of pain in my shoulder but nothing horrendous.

My belly is still swollen and hard but I'm sure that's from the gas still being trapped and not having been for a number 2 yet. So I will be on the Senna this evening that's for sure.

No bleeding, no leaking, nothing coming from me.

Still feeling mixed emotionally, I'm a bit narked at the doctor for not speaking to me properly afterwards and explaining a bit more what all this means for me 'cos obviously I've come away and Googled it – NOT a good idea.

I have learnt that due to the stress on your body of the op it can postpone OV so I'm going to order some OPKs today so I can monitor that.

It's weird that my skin has started to dry out, I don't have much of an appetite and I usually love my food but I'm hoping to get out and about today and maybe work up an appetite.

So all in all I feel good not great but not crap but good.

I hope that lasts all day.

20th June 2010
Lap & Dye: One Month on – TMI Warning

This month itself has been a mini roller coaster for me and I feel the need to let it out.

I have read that it's common to feel depressed after an op even one as small as a L&D but man I had no idea.

Physically: I have just had my AF, she was one day late and it was indeed different. There was no heavy onslaught as usual but it was painful. A different type of pain compared to what I'm used to. This was more a stabbing pain as opposed to the normal crampy, muscular type. I had to come out of the swimming pool 'cos it hurt so bad. The AF itself was light, it was more like EWCM mixed in, but it did contain an array of pin head sized clots. I only 'bled' for 2 days and now today it has been trailing off so to speak.

Psychologically: God I feel down and out. I feel like the world hates me, then I feel stupid for feeling like that so punish myself mentally for being so weak. Straight after the Lap I felt so positive and now it's gone. But it's gone way further than it's ever gone from me before. I know that my body is healing and I need to give it time, but how long is long enough?

My current thoughts are that if I ever manage to get my follow up appointment with the FS then I feel that she will tell me to go away for 6 months and see what happens. A few people are opposed to this theory and seem to think that because we have been TTC for so long they won't make me wait, but we'll see.

Having read as much as I have now read about my stage 2 endometriosis, I think I can put it into perspective.

The average couple have a 25% chance each cycle of conceiving, when you [I] have Mild Endo; those chances go down to 7% a cycle. So maybe, just maybe, the odds are now more in my favour.

So, I am now going to relax, there's nothing more I can do than I have already done.

I don't what to know what cycle day I am, I don't want to know when I'm due to ovulate, I just don't WANT to know anymore.

I will concentrate on my health and fitness and cut myself some bloody slack for a change.

It WILL happen – but unfortunately my crystal ball can't tell me when.

12th July 2010
Lap & Dye: The Next Step

It's been about 6 weeks since I had a Lap & Dye, and for those of you that don't know, they found Stage 2 Endometriosis.

I had my letter for my follow up appointment last week for this morning at 11.15, I took the day off work, made DH take a couple of hours off to come with me.

We arrived bang on time and emerged no more than 5 minutes later.

I am perfect, we are perfect.

I was sat down and was shown photographs of my ovaries, my tubes, my liver and the dye in them and of the Endo before they lasered them away.

My consultant was very happy with everything and after telling me this she said that for up to 4 months following the op, we have a 70% chance of achieving pregnancy. (She's telling me this with a big grin on her face as if she's handed me a BFP.)

I am ovulating (a big orange patch on my ovary showed her this), my tubes are clear, no more Endo and SA is good.

She said relax, take a holiday and have sex 'cos there's nothing stopping you now. If we're not [pregnant] in 4 months then come back but she's not expecting to see us again. The nurse even said as we were leaving to give them a ring to arrange things when 'it' happens.

I've had mixed feelings whilst dealing with this latest episode, but reading what I'm writing now and OMG, can this actually happen now?

Is that a hint of PMA I feel returning?

A wise person told me 'It's like learning Spanish with no tapes or books, you need the right equipment, and now you have the equipment you need'.

So I'm officially writing off the past *whispers* 3 and ½ years 'cos I didn't have the right tools, and a new outlook to getting our BFP pe (post endo) by October 2010.

I was Fran TTC 3.6 with Endo, I'm now Fran TTC 1 cycle pe.

20th August 2010
Pain after Endo Lap & Dye

It's been 3 months since the op and I'm still in pain.

I have a dull aching pain in my left side which can sometimes get quite intense and feel like a stabbing pain and it hurts so much I find myself pushing against it.

Also my back is in constant agony, I don't know if it's related or not and cannot find any further info on any of it. I think I will have to ring the FS office on Tuesday 'cos I can't keep living on paracetamol.

7th September 2010
My Next Step

With it just turning September, it dawned on me that we have to go back to the FS at the end of October so I've decided to go and give reflexology a good go.

Had a good chat with the lady that does it and we have put a plan in place for me which I'm looking forward to 'cos even if it doesn't help, it still really relaxes me which I think I need now.

I'm also finding myself very positive lately, and this is something I haven't felt for a very long time. I'm so positive that my AF will not show and I will get a bit of left over brown IB.

I am PG – I will have a BFP on Friday 10th of Sept – watch this space!

New house: new start: new family member.

5th October 2010
FS Appointment: 6 months Post Op

She basically said we have two options now because there's nothing wrong with us so she can't understand why we're not PG.

Option 1: IUI. She explained this to us (but I know already) about washing sperm, monitoring OV with scans and 'inseminating' (romantic, hey) me an hour after DH gives a sample.

Option 2: IVF. As of today, we are on the NHS waiting list, it's 12 months long. After pondering this I realised if we do end up having IVF it's going to be another two years before I get my LO; 1 year waiting, treatment then cooking, so although it's positive we're on there, I bloody well hope I don't have to wait that long.

She said we can do IUI whilst waiting for IVF if we want, DH perked up at this point and said, 'yes, whatever it takes!'

So that's what we're doing, had to sign a bunch of consent forms in front of the FS then went with the nurse into treatment room to go through details. I thanked the FS for all her help and went into the other room and burst out crying. The nurse hugged me and I told her I was gutted it had come to this. She said don't be down 'cos it's not over yet.

SO: she went through instructions, I'm on CD21 today so had progesterone bloods done to check my OV status, I have to go back between days 2–4 and have a selection of bloods done which DH had done today, then ring the nurse to arrange a scan for CD11 and every other day to monitor my follicles. When they're about to burst DH and I will come in, he will do his sample, they will wash it all and an hour later they will stick it in me.

I don't know what the success rates are; I'm probably going to scour boards for other experiences now.

En route back to car DH asked me to explain IUI to him again, so I did, and he laughed,

'so they'll get the best of the best boys then'.

He was fab today, again his attitude is whatever needs to be done he will do, it reminds me that he does want a family.

So all in all, I think that's what we expected, isn't it?

26th October 2010
IUI Step 1 CD11

Endometrium (lining of womb) is measuring at 6.6mm, it needs to be at least 8mm for PG and for IUI to continue so that's thickening nicely.

Left Ovary has 1 follicle measuring 10mm and right ovary has 2 follicles measuring 12mm and 13mm, I grew them all on my own.

I told her I've always suspected that my left side is weaker.

Anyway, FN (fertility nurse) was very happy with results and we discussed the next step. She was a bit hesitant that I would OV on weekend, I told her there was no chance as I am low on CBFM and tend to OV later in cycle anyway and she was happy with that. So after a good chat we've decided that next scan is 12pm on Monday, based on average growth rate and stuff we should be looking at Wednesday morning to DTD (lol).

As long as the scan is good on Monday, I will be shown how to inject myself Monday night between 10pm and 12am, this injection will ensure that eggy pops out and doesn't decide to sod off and give me an anovulatory cycle and put everything to cock. This injection takes 36 hours to work hence the Weds morning 'insemination' – LUSH word.

29th October 2010
IUI step 2 CD14

Scan booked for 12pm so off I toddle and get there a little early, about 11.45am, I don't get in until 12.15pm. Lovely scan ladies, I asked them for a guided tour (lol) which I had. Womb lining is 7.5mm which is fab as it has to be at least 8mm to sustain a bean. The left ovary still has a follicle which now only measures 7mm but there are lots of little ones there too.

Right ovary has a nice big juicy one at 16.5mm and again a few little ones so everything's looking great.

They fill in my form with all my details and I head off upstairs to see my nurse to go through it all and arrange next step...only to find there is no nurse. No-one to give my injection for tonight, no-one to arrange IUI on Weds morning: NO ONE. My main nurse is at home and has left her phone number in anticipation of my scan, the receptionist tries her 3 times whilst I'm there with no luck, goes to answer phone.

I get quite shirty at this point and explain to the receptionist what is supposed to be going on, I ask her to keep trying FN and left my mobile for her to contact me on.

GUTTED is an understatement.

So, I drive back to work (via McDonalds) a bit down, there's actually nothing I can do.

So I firstly ring my local hospital, this is where I believed that the IUI would be taking place not the hospital I've been frequenting (Port Talbot) only to be told that they have no record or notes of anything to do with me receiving IUI this week. Lady on phone was very apologetic and was gutted she couldn't help me when I explained to her my predicament.

So I ring my other FN (the one I cried on last week) who has been posted to another hospital (Swansea) and can't get hold of her. In a last ditch attempt I ring Port Talbot again only to be told by a recorded message that they're closed. That's it, no more I can do today. I'm very down about this right now, I've been so excited and everything has gone so smoothly until this.

So I will ring the PT hospital in the morning and try again to speak to someone 'cos TBH I don't really know what else I can do. I don't wanna go BDing in case we still have the IUI this week as we have to abstain but also know there's eggys growing and don't want to miss my chance. Sorry for the long one, another day in my TTC rollercoaster ride.

30th October 2010
IUI Step 3 CD15

After yesterday's shocking display of NHS services, I rang first thing this morning when they opened to be told there was nobody in to speak to and that I should phone back tomorrow when my FN nurse is in.

I was very, very tamping.

Still only 'high' on CBFM.

Climbed back into bed and the phone rang, Nurse Sharon returning my call wanting me to go get scanned today based on yesterday's results.

Apparently my FN did get in touch with the ward but it wasn't passed down to me. I thanked her profusely and was booked in for 12pm. Went along and it's the same radiologist that scanned me yesterday so we had a natter whilst having a rummage.

My womb lining (endometrium) is still only 7.8mm, 7.5 yesterday and needs to be 8mm. Left ovary still the same and one great big follicle on the right ovary measuring a lovely 18.5mm. So the folly's fine but they will not proceed with treatment if the lining doesn't thicken enough so I am back down tomorrow morning at 8.30 for ANOTHER scan.

The lining increased by 0.3mm in exactly 24hrs so I'm hoping it will thicken by 0.2mm by 2moro morning. As long as it has, it's all systems go, I don't know what go means just yet but as soon as I do you will. By the way it's my FN on duty tomorrow morning so I hope she isn't shitty with me 'cos she'll be getting chinned.

31st October 2010
IUI Step4 CD16

8.30am scan this morning, in there early to ensure I'm first one in. My lovely lining is measuring at 9.8mm and right follicle is a whopping 20mm – we're good to go. Upstairs to the ward I go to see our FN who apologises for my shocking treatment on Monday. She rings local hospital to arrange the IUI, it's booked to 9am semen deposit on CD18. She gives me my injection of Ovitrelle and explains how to administer at 9pm that night wishes me luck and sends me on my merry way. I am very, very excited and making a baby Friday morning.

2nd November 2010
IUI Final Step CD18

Didn't sleep for most of the night, a bit like a kid on Xmas eve.

Very, very excited for what today would bring, one step closer to my BFP. DH does his bit at 8.45am and off we go, tub between my boobies to keep them cosy and down to the hospital for 9am. Arrived and parked, and suddenly realised we've not completed any of the paperwork we were given so take a pen in with us. We're the first ones there and the nurse takes us into a room to start the ball rolling.

We produce our driving licences and fill in the paperwork. We hand over the boys ready for their scrubbing and are told to return at 9.45am for my turn!

Eeekkkk!

Cuppa tea time and I prepare to get my fadge out again. Half an hour later at 9.45 we return and tell them we're back, at 10.05 we're still waiting and I find myself saying 'I hope nothing's wrong'. 5 minutes later we're called and grinning like kids we go in.

'I'm very sorry to tell you we can't continue with the IUI.

There's not enough sperm in the sample to continue!'

I will remember that split second for eternity.

I remember asking to see the results; there were only 6 million before washing and only 250,000 afterwards. The nurse asked about the last SA and I told her the count was 50 million so off she went to look for some notes on that. When we were left in the room I took DHs hand and he said, 'At least it's not you', he was white and mortified and I cried. Not a huge sobbing cry but enough tears to notice.

We were left 10 minutes until she came back with the last SA results which was back in [last] January. Why don't they check the men more regularly? The amount I've had done to me surely it would make sense? The FS in that hospital wants DH to go back on the 22nd of November and do another test. They're very hopeful it's just a blip 'cos the last one was fine.

God, we're devastated.

I feel like I've completely let him down, it's been about me with B12, EPO, reflexology and that poor bugger's got shite swimmers! That all happened a couple of days ago and it's taken me this long to get my head round it and deal with it. We've got the Wellman/woman conception tablets and I've bought Zita West's fertility book which I'm going through and am going to make my DH my number one priority. I'm not hoping for miracles in 3 weeks but I am hoping to get those boys dancing.

9th December 2010
Where Have I Been?

I have felt so lost, so lost. I haven't felt like myself. I've been down and in a funk. I have been constantly anxious and depressed. Man, I've been so down.

I know it's just a case of sorting my head out and now I think I've finally done it.

Since our f***ed up IUI attempt and my poor hubby's face that day, it destroyed me. I felt so bad, I've forked out £100 for him to get a tattoo.

I never want him to feel like that again.

It's CD2 today, and 2 days ago my niece turned 2, and I remember when SIL texted me to tell me she was PG and I remember thinking 'Bollox, she beat me to it' that was nearly 3 years ago when you take a pregnancy into account. F**K – where'd my life go?

AF is painful today, reminds me of AF pre-L&D and figure the endo is creeping back and we know the only cure is a PG right?

I was reading my paperwork from the London Women's Clinic yesterday and I smiled, there's a 50% chance that our 1st IVF cycle will work.

50% is good freaking odds to me.

I smiled, and smiled at everything, at all the questions and realised that yes, this is going to happen and yes, I will be PG in 2011.

May not have been the way I envisioned it to happen but sometimes Mother Nature needs a helping hand.

So I have a plan – I have 2 cycles before D-day. This cycle OV is literally over Xmas and next cycle will be a weekend.

So I have some EPO for extra CM and will be dusting off the CBFM but still having lots of fun regular sex with DH on his 'man-vits'.

The race to the 1st 2011 BFP begins – and I intend to win.

9th February 2011
Initial IVF Consultant Appointment

Arrived at 1.30, all paperwork handed in and I had my scan and DH done another SA.

2.45pm we get into the Dr's office.

She explains that Welsh Assembly Government guidelines state that the one year wait is mandatory for NHS funded IVF. I expected this. She explained that we would get 2 full IVF cycles and 2 FETs so you could really count it as four goes.

She goes through a ream of questions about everything imaginable for DH and me.

After that, she said that there's nothing more we could do, but had I heard of Egg Sharing? To which I said, yes, I've read about it. She said that if this is something I would be willing to do then I would qualify for a free private cycle with them.

She was very surprised when I said that I would be willing to do it.

She runs through a few things and explains that if SA comes back low again then we would need ICSI, which she explains is NOT free and would need to be paid for as a supplement along with the HFEA fee.

I'm not going to even worry about that right now. It could come back that my bloods are rubbish, or I have a chromosomal defect or something then we're not even going to get that far.

So I had my AMH (whatever that is) blood taken and sent off and I will be ringing to find results of that on Friday.

According to the letter which I received today (fast or what) if all results are satisfactory then they will be looking to begin the Egg Sharing cycle immediately. Fancy that, hey?

I am CD7 today, I'm wondering if it would be as fast as next cycle?

Best get back on Slimming World to make sure my BMI doesn't creep back up and scupper my plans.

I am making eggs for 2 now after all. Smug or what?

10th March 2011
Heartbroken

I'm in such an odd place right now.

I feel like such a failure for not being able to make a baby. I look at people every day with their babies, bumps or LOs, and always wonder why not me?

I have so much to be thankful for, I feel so ungrateful and selfish for wanting 'one more thing'.

I want my son, I want my husband's little baby boy that sometimes I cry so much at my own disappointment.

I want his BFP, I want to feel his first kick, I want to decorate his room and buy him all new stuff. I want to birth him with DH by my side and take him home all safe and sound.

I want to change his smelly nappy and worry about whether I BF or FF, I want to take him round to family houses for Sunday lunches where everyone fusses him. I want to take him into work and show off this little creation that we made. I want to hear him wake at night and go comfort him 'cos I'm his Mummy and that's my job.

I want to see him smile, and play and crawl. I want to see him grow and buy him his first pair of Clarks. I want to see him running around pulling the dog's ears and hiding Daddy's tools.

Do I now finally want my son so much that we can make it happen?

How after all this time can I still think we will get our miracle and I can cancel IVF?

I want him, I want him so much I could scream and cry and stamp my feet 'til I get him.

One day soon he will be ours...

7th April 2011
Acceptance

It's been 6 months since being put on the list for IVF (in Wales there's a mandatory one year wait).
It's taken this long for me to accept that we need treatment.

What a hard realisation.

I've still wondered and hoped that we'll still get our miracle natural BFP but after nearly 4 and a half years, who am I kidding, right?

So this will be my last AT cycle until I begin ICSI in October.

No more CBFM, OPKs or anything. I will keep taking the EPO 'cos it stops my boobies hurting from OV to AF!

I'm going to actually stop TTC; I will put my energy and focus into passing my exams in May, turning 30 in June, and then moving into our new home in July and all the while losing my last stone of weight.

I want to have sex when I'm horny and not because I have to.

I want to stop begrudging my husband 'cos he has a lower sex drive than me and doesn't wanna DTD all the time (quality rather than quantity hey?).

So I've finally accepted that it's ICSI for us. BFP in October, anyone gonna join me?

16th June 2011
It's my 30th Birthday

And it's a bitter sweet day.

AF is due Saturday and I was secretly hoping for a miracle B'day BFP but to no avail.

I thought I would've had my first baby by 30, but it was not meant to be.

Don't get me wrong, I'm not sad, and this is not a 'downer' journal, but merely another milestone marker.

I know this will be my last B'day not being a Mummy. ICSI in October will work and I should be due around this time next year (ish).

I don't know how I feel, I feel lucky to have accomplished many things and am excited for everything to come.

It's been such a long journey; I hope we're blessed with a sticky SullyBug soon to complete our family.

Every day is a milestone and a day closer to our dreams coming true.

16th August 2011
The Final Countdown

Time for an update, I feel.

It's August, there are 10 days until we move home (we've been at MILs for 7 months) and then we start prep for IVF, which is redoing bloods and ordering my drugs.

I've had a read back over my past few journals and laughed and cried at them; but I have stuck to my words, I've not TTC'd for many, many cycles, no CBFM, no OPKs nothing, I've just got on with my life and it's been quite nice.

There's so much that's about to happen in my life, and I'm so scared and excited all in the same bundle.

I have seen many, many BFPs and births over the past 6 months, many of whom I have been so, so ecstatic for and others have had me wondering, 'Why you and not me, you haven't been at it as long' or other such bonkers thoughts. I've seen families break up and children get caught in the middle of rows, and thought, 'Why did you deserve to have that child and not me?'

I still have the crazy, jealous thoughts and feelings, but in no way the same way as I used to. I'm actually quite embarrassed at some of the stuff I wrote, but I know that at the time that was my world, and that's how I felt.

With approximately 6 weeks to go before we start IVF, I am so excited to finally get pregnant, so gutted that's it come to this, and so incredibly overwhelmed with dreams and plans for the future.

Won't be long SullyBug, Mummy and Daddy are coming to get you.

9th September 2011
My ICSI Journey

I think it will be easier in the long run if I record this journey in one entry and just update accordingly.

26th of August
Just moved into our new home and today is the day we go to the clinic to get our bloods redone.

Whilst we're there, I chat with the nurse about start date. I figure we've waited near enough a year and having to wait until CD1 in October was a bit mean and she agreed. So we will be starting CD1 end of September which should work out about the 17th. We update our records with new home address and she orders my drugs and tells me to ring CD1.

Monday 5th of September
My drugs arrived this morning in a box!

There's loads of them and it completely spun me out! I did not realise there would be so much to take. DH said he looked forward to injecting me (sadistic sod) and then I come across the power progesterone suppositories! They are to be taken rectally from EC until ET and then they can be administered VAGINALLY! He said he wouldn't be helping with those! LOL.

So that's it, all ready to go, roll on CD1.

Thursday 8th of September
Getting IVF cold feet today! Wondering if it hasn't happened for a reason and perhaps we're not meant to have kids and it's just not meant to be. Yikes.

Friday 9th of September
Cold feet fading, added another name to my 'list' today, felt a bit better. Had a light bit of spotting, only CD23, wondering if AF will show herself early so we can get on with things?!

Tuesday 13th September
Feeling excited again today. I can feel AF knocking; I just hope my bloods are back at the clinic, think I'll give them an email to check.

Odd to think this time next week I'll be 'stimming' my eggs. Eeekk!

Still having the 1 or 2 embie debate in my head.

2pm: screening blood tests are back and we are good to go. AF due Friday, hopefully she arrives on time as the clinic isn't open on weekends. Woo hoo! Here we go.

Thursday 15th September
AF came at 11am, rang clinic now at 12.30pm, baseline scan booked for Saturday 17th at 8.30am.

Saturday 17th September (CD2)
Arrived at clinic, pants off and on the bed, couldn't find my right ovary, took a lot of prodding and poking but she was there with 3 follies, my left ovary was another story. There was a massive follie there. Explains so much with my cycle, constant OV pain in the left side 'cos it seems I'm constantly OVing, but then so many questions; why has this not been picked up before? Do I OV straight after AF and then the LH surge mid cycle is a fake? Or have I been OVing twice? If it's the latter then God don't I have rubbish timing and luck!

So, after consulting with the doctor, I have been put on Microgynon BC for 21 days to kill off the follies and start from scratch, so more or less on Long Protocol now.

Just hoping it doesn't take ages for AF to come when I've finished taking them.

Yet another curve ball hey?

sigh

Friday 23rd September (CD8)
Weekly update time, only 14 pills left, yey! They are making me nauseous which is pants, but I suppose I better get used to it. I'm sure between the DR drugs and the stimms I will be feeling sick enough and then morning sickness will kick in so I'll just get used to it.

I'm not online much anymore, which is partly through choice and partly being too busy, but TBH

I've found I'm so much more chilled out. Putting quality time into our new home and just relaxing is great. Going to give my new running app a whirl in the morning. Tomorrow will only be 13...

4th October 2011
My ICSI Journey Part 2

Can't believe I only have 3 pills left to take. I'm hoping to be back in the clinic this time next week. I'm so scared of something else happening though and setting us back. I'm so sick of fighting for everything. I want to get excited and look forward but we didn't even get past the first scan. I'm normally usually such an optimistic person, I can visualise things and stay focused but this IVF stuff is such unknown territory.

My little bit of PMA this week was used to order myself the iCandy brochure.

Hope for the best but prepare for the worst, one day at a time

Thursday 6th of October 2011
Tomorrow is my last pill! Get those pom poms out, I hope this AF is here ASAP and is really heavy and flushes everything out, I don't want any little follies left in there after what has been the LONGEST 21 days!

It occurred to me that a year ago yesterday we were put on the IVF waiting list, that we took a leap of faith and left our home of 7 years. A leap of faith; that's what it has been all along, is a leap of faith.

Faith...George Michael had it and God damn it I gotta have faith that ICSI will work and in 4 weeks times I will be getting my first ever BFP, and it will be sticky and squishy and will result in Sullybug next July. See you in 10 months, baby.

Monday 10th of October 2011
Still no bloody witch! Aarrggh lol! First time ever I've wanted her to turn up and she's messing with me! Last pill was Friday morning so I'm hoping

any day now. Although just checking my app and my regular AF would be due this Saturday anyways.

I'm kind of in limbo a little today, been asked to go out for Halloween and host parties but TBH I think I've got enough to concentrate on without stretching myself to compensate others.

I'll just have to play the miserable bitch card until I get my BFP then everyone will understand!

Just getting loads of EWCM now with brown so hopefully she'll show up soon enough.

Wednesday 12th October 2011 – CD1
Witch here, scan tomorrow, bricking it. But did indulge in a little Mothercare perusal whilst in town. Not done that in a VERY long time. 27 hours and counting...

15th October 2011
ICSI Part Trois

CD4 today, Day 3 of DR Supercur (200ml) and Day 2 of Gonal F(300ml)

Feeling good, and positive. Actually I probably feel the best I have in a very long time.

DH is loving giving me the jabs bless him; deffo makes him feel part of the action and keeping us together through this.

Frigg I'm just so excited but realistic as well that if everything doesn't work out then back to my bubble I go. But it's irrelevant, because I know it's going to work, there's not a doubt in my mind than in 24 days' time I will have my VERY LONG awaited 1st ever BFP, and how there will be an extra special Christmas present for all the family this year.

19th October 2011
CD9, just done injections and they hurt. Belly feels like it's going to burst.

Booked some leave from work next week for what will hopefully be EC and then ET.

Can't wait to get to this scan on Friday now to see if everything's ok.

Not really sure what happens after that.

Another day done.

24th October 2011
Lucky No 7 ICSI Part 4
What a wild ride of emotions this past week has been.

Had my EC this morning and they recovered 7 eggs from 7 follicles. I'm so over the freaking moon with that, my second over the moon moment came when I learnt that DH's SA is now in the 'normal' range!

So proof that you can get the stats up.

We will still be having (would've been done by now) ICSI. OMG that's so crazy to think that my babies are cultivating in a petri dish. OK so I'm sure it's a bit more advanced than that but you get the drift.

I'm not greedy; one great embie will make me over the moon, anything over that is a bonus.
I've not been this excited at the prospect of having a baby for such a long time I can't remember.

Had a browse at some stuff online and wondering if I finally get to buy some stuff.

I've planned how I'm going to tell everyone. Yes, yes I'm crazy I know, but PMAing it up like you wouldn't believe right now.

It's been decided whether they're boys or girls, what DNA they have, who they will look like, our babies were conceived today.

So cwtch down little embies, grow strong for us, I can't wait to hear how you're doing in the morning.

Good night babies, grow well.

6th November 2011
The end of one chapter begins with another.

Nothing else to say right now.

Update from Amy (July 2013)

Of course I couldn't just leave it there!

In June 2012 Fran gave birth to twin boys.

Due to the position of the babies (one breech, one transverse) she was booked in for a Caesarean Section at 38 weeks. However, two weeks before this she went into labour naturally and the boys were delivered via an emergency C-section. Both of them spent time in the SCBU but soon came home.

A year on they are healthy, happy, energetic little boys.

You can read her full birth story on page 192.

Chapter 5

Telling the world

It's a very personal decision about when and how to share the news of your pregnancy. Given the popularity and use of social media, a common method is to simply post a scan picture for all to admire and comment. Since the 12 week point (and dating scan) signals a 'safer' milestone in the pregnancy calendar, many choose to wait until this has passed before spreading their news.

I will admit I found it difficult to keep our secret until the 12 week mark. My sister was the first to know, followed closely by the rest of our families. We did wait until we had had our scan before divulging to our friends and although they were not shocked, it came as a lovely surprise.

How did your friends and family react to your pregnancy news?

Family and friends were very excited. A couple of friends back home found it tough as I didn't live near them and felt a little jealous because it was hard to share the experience with them. (Em)

'I guessed that you were pregnant. You weren't drinking and it's not like you to turn down a glass of wine!' (Kate)

Mostly surprise. A few people were really excited on my behalf – some Uni friends and, bizarrely, my dad who I had been dreading telling! My other close friends didn't know what to think really. My boyfriend's family were quite worried. They barely knew me and were worried for him and how it would affect him/his future. (Kathy)

My boss shouted it out to the whole office when I told him, the whole office cheered and shouted, it was lovely! Mum and Dad were over the moon as it would be their first grandchild and Dom's Mum was over the moon too (her second grandchild). All of our friends were delighted too! Many of our friends have kids so they were excited that another was coming along. (Lindsay)

Surprise from both sides of the family. We hadn't told them we were trying (or had miscarried) so they just assumed we didn't want children. (Beth)

Everyone was ecstatic. I had been public about my previous loss and I knew people knew we had been trying since we got married so they were all saying we deserved it and they were very happy for us. When I phoned my best friend to tell her she first told me that she had just suffered a miscarriage, we would have been due the same time. Her first thoughts on being pregnant were feelings of dread regarding how she would tell me. I felt really bad about this. I then told her our news and we had a bit of a cry about the whole bitter sweetness of the situation. (Jane)

Everyone was very excited although I was most shocked by my partner's brother who was very interested in my pregnancy. It was really sweet; he even had a pregnancy app on his iPhone and would fill me in on what were the week's developments (although I already knew!) He was on birth watch from about 38 weeks making sure he wasn't getting drunk and had a car to get to the hospital if needed. (Claire)

Mostly positive: it did change my relationship with my bestie significantly in that we no longer had our long nights out drinking, although it just means a different relationship now. As I got pregnant so quickly it put significant pressure on my new colleague to learn the job quickly (there are only two of us) which was not ideal for her, although she has been very supportive! (Jessica)

We had told our close family first time round about being pregnant so after the miscarriage they knew we were trying for a baby. Everyone was so happy for us when they found out we were pregnant again. When I told people at work a few people said they had guessed and when we told friends we got the same reaction.

My friends from York found out they were pregnant at the same time as us (3 weeks ahead) and waited to tell us on my friend's birthday at her birthday meal to a response of 'Oh my God, so are we'. It was really nice to be pregnant at the same time especially with my friend being a few weeks ahead as she could reassure me that there was pregnancy beyond feeling sick. My friend was also able to share experiences about maternity appointments and she had a few bleeds in the first trimester and went on to have a problem-free pregnancy so she helped to reassure me that I wasn't going to have another miscarriage. (Emma)

A lot of people were very surprised as we have never been 'children' people but everyone was happy for us. My in-laws were particularly pleased as they thought we would never have children and my husband is an only child. My mother-in-law was quite resentful that we wouldn't give her grandchildren so she was over the moon. A couple of people said that we'd never cope and were quite sceptical but it's been fun proving them wrong. (Christie)

People were generally very excited but suddenly I became a fragile being. I couldn't pick anything up, reach anywhere, do anything without someone rushing to help. (Natalie)

We found being told 'well done' strange. I loved the attention from strangers and always smiled at people in the street, more than usual. We had lots of warning about this being the end of our lives and 'you wait and see' type stuff thrown at our optimism and certainty we'd be happy, just as free, and that the baby wouldn't be a devil child. (Jenna)

The most predominant impression was 'finally'. When the complications arose I got encouragement from lots of people who said that they were praying for us. Generally, everyone was sharing in the joy. (Cheryl)

I had some lovely reactions on being pregnant from friends and family. The best was telling my close work colleagues on a girly night around mine before Christmas. There were so many screams and hugs!

I told my mum and dad over Skype as they were going away for the weekend before we were telling Pete's parents. My dad was dancing around and my mum was ecstatic. Of course I did get the comments on already suffering from baby brain! (Lou)

My and my husband's parents were over the moon that we were finally having a child! (Zoe)

Chapter 6

The first trimester

Calculating due-dates and how far along you are in your pregnancy can be quite confusing.

The given '9 months' gestation for a typical pregnancy is actually calculated as 40 weeks from the date of your last period: your doctor or midwife will give you an estimated due date based on the date of your last period.

These 40 weeks are then divided into three trimesters: the first trimester is weeks 1 to 13; the second trimester is weeks 14 to 27 and the third trimester is weeks 27 to 40.

The first trimester can be a real rollercoaster of emotions. Your hormones are going crazy, you often need to pee multiple times throughout the night; sometimes you are sick or just feel like you have a constant hangover! Many women report on the overwhelming tiredness that hits in this trimester. And of course most people keep their pregnancy a secret until their dating scan (between 8 and 14 weeks) so find it difficult hiding their sickness from friends and family.

How did you feel during the first trimester?

Sick and tired! Also very scared after losing a baby previously, this made me very nervous and I didn't really enjoy the first part of my pregnancy as I was so paranoid. (Claire)

Fine, some sick feelings during the late afternoon, but otherwise fine. I was cautious as I had experienced miscarriage in the first trimester so was aware of not getting too excited until I had had the first scan. (Vicki)

Very tired and a bit nauseous but nothing awful. (Rachel)

Tired! I had three jobs at the time as it was the university summer holidays. I also had morning sickness so my morning job in a canteen with the smells of food was not very pleasant. However I developed a very strong attachment to my little one during this time. (Kathy)

I was fine, didn't feel very different apart from not wanting to eat much. I went off chocolate and couldn't finish my dinner which is VERY unlike me. Smells were a lot stronger though and I went off a hand cream I usually used and couldn't be near a smoker at work. Apart from that I had no sickness which I was so happy about. (Lou)

I was extremely nervous as I wanted to know the baby was okay. I felt very tired and nauseous, yet was never actually sick. I did have two early bleeds at 5 and 8 weeks which was very scary in which I had early scans. I had a kidney infection as well which was very painful too. I couldn't wait to have a bump to show it off. (Em)

Fine, a little nauseous now and again but no actual sickness. I felt tired, but then always did going to work anyway so no real difference! I had a little spotting for a few days which was a worry, but it was nothing. I got a urine infection but a week of antibiotics cleared it. It completely zaps all your energy for a week or so, I took time off work for it and slept loads. (Lindsay)

It was like I had constant motion sickness and was really tired. (Laura)

Tired, tea tasted weird and I started craving orange juice like there was no tomorrow. (Beth)

Not too bad all in all. I didn't suffer too badly from morning sickness. I did feel a bit queasy quite often, but if I ate something then it passed. I used to go round with bagfuls of apples in my bag. Fortunately I had only recently moved offices at work, so no one noticed that I had suddenly started snacking quite a lot. I completely went off tea and coffee, so my drink of choice became hot water. The only time that I was really sick was when we went on holiday abroad. I think that it was just the fact that I was eating slightly different food to usual, and not necessarily what I really wanted. For a number of days in a row I went down to breakfast and then as soon as I started to eat anything I had to rush quickly back to our room to be sick. I didn't suffer from tiredness too badly, but I did get really thirsty at night so I had to drink gallons of water, and then of course had to keep going to the toilet. (Kate)

Fine – a bit more tired but no sickness, etc. (Louisa)

Until the first scan I was convinced the tests were wrong. I was really lucky, apart from going off peppermint tea and finding I needed 8 hours sleep to function, I had no symptoms. I was excited that my husband and I had our little secret. I really looked forward to telling our immediate family as he was a much wanted first grandchild on both sides. I decided that I wanted the kitchen replaced and the nursery needed re-plastering all before the baby arrived. (Zoe)

Petrified that something could go wrong but except for an aversion to poultry and poultry products, there were no signs or symptoms. (Cheryl)

I felt nauseous all the time but was only actually sick on a handful of occasions.
Nothing really helped – I tried ginger snaps as recommended by other people and my doctor but I grew to really dislike them as the smell of them reminded me of feeling sick (this wore off after I gave birth).
I also started using a lemon fragranced body cream to prevent stretch marks and the smell of lemons even now reminds me of feeling sick. I was also nervous and looked forward to reaching my second trimester as I knew the risk of having a miscarriage significantly reduces.
I was very tired and would often fall asleep on the sofa after tea. (Emma)

I felt panicky a lot about losing the baby. I had a scan at under five weeks which didn't show the pregnancy in the womb, blood tests were done and the results were good but it was an agonising wait to see if the embryo had implanted in the right place. Then after we found that out we had more early scans to show a heartbeat. It was amazing and scary all at once. I was a nervous pregnant woman who needed masses of support to be reassured that the chances of losing this pregnancy was small. (Jane)

Awful: all day morning sickness, constant nausea and migraines but I found the stomach pains reassuring and couldn't wait to use a Doppler at home and feel kicking. (Jenna)

I was very sick pretty much from day one and it would last all day. I was also very emotional and cried at everything. It was like having crazy bad PMT for 14 weeks!

I also found it very hard because I wasn't supposed to be telling anyone and it was so difficult to hide all my symptoms. I was also exhausted. I would actually fall asleep at my desk.

Oh, and I started peeing every 10 minutes from about week 5 and that didn't stop until after the baby was born.

I didn't have the same worries about miscarriage as a lot of others though because I was part of a trial in London so I got a scan at 6 weeks, 8 weeks and 10 weeks, which kept me reassured that everything was fine. (Christie)

Chapter 7

Advice

I found that as soon as people knew I was pregnant they couldn't help but impart advice – welcome or otherwise. Most of it was well meaning; some of it I ignored and some I wish I had taken more notice of. So-called 'Old Wives' Tales' and out-dated schools of thought have a lot to answer for; but there *are* also genuine causes for concern – so please listen to the health professionals.

What advice did you receive? (and did you take any notice?!)

'Put your feet up' – I ignored this and didn't feel any ill effects.

'Enjoy your maternity leave before the baby comes and don't do too much' – also ignored and maybe slightly regret that one now...! (Vicki)

My tutor at university suggested I didn't continue with the pregnancy – his advice was that I had a bright future and still had so much of the world to see and things to do and none of that would come if I had the baby. I'd already made up my mind by then though (I was a little over three months) so his words didn't have any effect. (Kathy)

Everyone had something to suggest but I did a lot of reading and so just ignored most of what people said that didn't correspond to my research. I did get some helpful tips on combatting morning sickness, though. Gingerbread men was the best for me (although I can't even look at one now!) (Christie)

I suppose take it easy as I did pretty much carry on up to about 30 weeks before I started to feel unwell. (Em)

Lots of mums told me to do my pelvic floor exercises which I tried, but never did them as much as I should! My mum told me not to reach up as it would get the umbilical cord wrapped around the baby's neck (this, it turns out, is a commonly believed Old Wives' Tale). (Laura)

My mum gave me lots of advice – more about how to deal with things myself rather than specific baby tips; like making sure my partner and I made time for each other and putting in regimented bedtimes (best advice ever) as soon as practical so I had 'non-mum' time in the day too. (Kathy)

It was useful having the monthly group on Baby Centre in terms of knowing other people's experiences and tips, I probably didn't take that much from people at home as I didn't know any other recent mums. (Jessica)

I ignored a lot from my mother-in-law who thinks pregnant people shouldn't do anything but be wrapped in bubble wrap and put in a box. (Beth)

'Don't eat peanut butter' – ignored! I felt it better to expose my baby to as much variety as possible and as no one in my family has a nut allergy I felt it safe enough. I also ate prawns from time to time when I know others told me not too and my egg yolks were sometimes a little runny! (Lindsay)

Advice taken: Listen to your body. Everyone has their own different pregnancy so don't worry if something is happening to someone else that isn't happening to you. (Natalie)

I only got well-meaning and non-intrusive advice from friends and family thankfully. I mainly took the advice of taking it easy, eating well and not stressing out about little things. I didn't go overboard on giving up food/drink as I had the odd glass of wine and still ate prawns and tuna. I didn't want to make it into a massive deal, although I was careful. (Lou)

Chapter 8

Mel's journey

I was keen for Mel to share her pregnancy journey as it seems such a rare phenomenon for a woman to experience. Mel suffers from Tocophobia – a fear of pregnancy and childbirth. For someone who suffers from this fear to even consider carrying a child is a terrifying prospect and Mel is the first to admit she struggled to come to terms with becoming a parent.

There is very little published research on Tocophobia in the UK and as such finding the statistics for how many women this affects is difficult. Many women request a C-section as a result of their phobia because of the fear of pain in childbirth.

Health authorities will deal with individual cases in accordance with their own guidelines, so if you have any concerns please contact your doctor or health professional.

'So this is me: I have Primary Tocophobia; yes, it has a name. This phobia is very embarrassing as a woman: all women want to have children right? Not in my case. The thought of growing one repulsed me, the thought of having a baby made me sick. It was so bad that I could not even look at a picture of a pregnant woman. If I walked into a supermarket and a pregnant woman was walking in at the same time I would have to start my shopping at the other end.

My phobia started in my teens. I had always been a tomboy and never ever wanted children, so much so that when I started being intimate, I took the pill and used condoms. When I was 21 I asked if I could be sterilised; thank God now they said no.

Then my body clock kicked in. I always said it wouldn't but it did!

All I wanted was a child, but that meant growing one, how the hell was I going to do that?

For a "normal" person, perhaps suffering something more common – such as arachnophobia – it would be like being in a tank full of spiders for 9 months.

So how did I get through my pregnancy with Colby? It started way before he was even here, 3 years in fact. I got help by using CBT (Cognitive Behavioural Therapy) and mindfulness training; these are used in a lot of phobias. I went once a month for 2 years before we even started trying: it's not easy and I had to work hard at it. When I did fall pregnant I did think 'how the hell am I going to get through this?' – however, this pregnancy was not meant to be. It was hard dealing with the miscarriage and I felt this was my doing because of the phobia. It was all in my head.

We started trying again after 3 months and bang, Colby was conceived and again the fun began. It still felt that I was growing a parasite, but with the therapy I could get my head around it. Going onto online chat rooms was a life-saver, because here I could be open and honest. I even managed a meet up in London, but asked that everyone covered up, which they did. I did not make the second meet because the ladies wouldn't be able to hide the bumps.

Talking to people was a must and Colby helped out a bit, I did not feel him move until 20 weeks due to the placenta being at the front. The midwife was very understanding and I had all my appointments first thing in the morning so there were not a lot of women in the waiting room. I had hoped to have a home birth but due to very high blood pressure it was not meant to be. Again, they were great in the hospital and I had my own room.

Would I do it again? No, I have got my little man, but it took a lot of mindfulness to have him and it was very draining.

Am I over the phobia? No, I just have the tools to work with it now.'

Chapter 9

Odd symptoms

There is a multitude of 'Old Wives' Tales' about your blooming body throughout pregnancy. For example, the different foods you crave are said to be an indicator of the sex of your baby: sweet food for a boy, sour or savoury for a girl.

My first-trimester nausea saw various cravings including one week of Skips crisps and apple juice and another week of sushi and orange juice. Mostly I just ate bread and butter, though.

Here are some of the cravings or odd symptoms that our Mums-to-be experienced during their pregnancies.

I didn't have any cravings – as popular media so often puts across – until around 6 months, when I suddenly only wanted to eat Mulligatawny Soup (which I haven't had since I was a child); just for a weekend, mind. Also, I no longer like gin and tonic, but do like whisky, having not done so before. (Jessica)

Hugely heightened sense of smell in the first trimester was very strange. (Laura)

No really weird ones for me. I was surprised how much I cried at everything though. (Christie)

Creme Egg cravings and tomato soup cravings. (Claire)

A complete aversion to my boyfriend's smell! Not very good for bonding. (Kathy)

The hair on my legs stopped growing – quite useful, since I wouldn't have been able to bend down to remove it towards the end! (Kate)

Hatred of all poultry products, including eggs. Eating or smelling such led to throwing up. (Cheryl)

It wasn't the oddest but I was addicted to beans and bagels and bags of crisps. (Em)

Probably the numb fingers; everything else was pretty standard text book. (Lindsay)

A craving for Bran Flakes.... (Vicki)

All of my sticky-out moles doubled in size: no one warns you of these kinds of things. (Natalie)

I didn't have many odd things just ferocious hunger where I would have to eat every hour in the first trimester. (Jane)

Had a month of almost only eating pepperoni pizza! (Rachel)

I went off eggs throughout my whole pregnancy. I couldn't bear to eat them or see anyone else eat them it made me feel really sick. I also went off cheese throughout the first 5 months of my pregnancy, but this wore off. (Emma)

Going off chocolate and really hating Lloyd Grossman pasta sauces (which I previously adored!!). I'm back on both now. (Lou)

I didn't really have any pregnancy symptoms. (Zoe)

Chapter 10

Plain sailing

I cannot reiterate or emphasise this enough – if you think anything is wrong during your pregnancy, go straight to your midwife or doctor. I wanted to share these examples of pregnancy problems to show how common they can be; but please do not use them to self-diagnose. Admittedly I had a fairly straightforward pregnancy, for which I am very thankful, but some of our Mums weren't as lucky.

Did you have any problems during your pregnancy?

I had a kidney infection and the most awful toothache. Although these were not scares as such, I wouldn't take painkillers so they were definitely problems! (Kathy)

I had a very quiet baby – didn't feel any movement until 26 weeks, and then probably only once a day after that, so I had some extra monitoring – all fine. No other problems. (Jessica)

Nope, text book pregnancy. She was transverse up until 31weeks but managed to turn with a lot of ball bouncing. She never engaged (not even when [my] waters broke) during the pregnancy but this didn't cause any problems. (Beth)

Two bleeds at 5 and 8 weeks and pre-eclampsia which was undetected until I went into labour at just under 37 weeks. (Em)

Only at the very end. A week before my due date the baby's movements slowed down significantly so I went in to be monitored for a few hours. (Laura)

I had reduced movement around 30 weeks so went to be scanned and monitored – glad they did as they found out maggot was breech! (Vicki)

Just the spotting in the 1st trimester which was fine (only lasted a day or two). Then urine infections and being sent to hospital with the glucose in my urine. (Lindsay)

The second time I had early bleeding so needed a 6 week scan. It felt quite scary waiting for it as a miscarriage was quite possible. (Rachel)

Gestational diabetes. Ugh, that diet was a nightmare! And related to that they said that baby would be big because of the GD, but she was actually one of the smaller babies of the group. That worried me for nothing. (Christie)

My little baby was breech and didn't turn. (Natalie)

I was referred to the hospital a few times by the midwife. The first was because I hadn't felt the baby move over the weekend. The baby's heart rate was monitored and everything was fine. Even though I felt like I had wasted their time the hospital staff were lovely and assured me they always preferred to check. The further two times were due to my bump measuring small. The hospital re-scanned to check the size of the baby and the amount of fluid. The second set of scans showed that I had low fluid and they decided to induce me the next day, a week before my due date, if a sweep didn't bring labour on. (Zoe)

Someone crashed into the back of my car when I was seven months pregnant which was pretty harrowing. It wasn't at a fast speed but it still shook me up. I went to the Midwife to get checked up the next day and the baby was fine. (Lou)

The initial period where we wondered would this baby have found its way to my womb or get stuck along the way. My sister told me I never referred to it as a baby until I had the scan at 7 weeks and saw the heartbeat. I hadn't realised this but she was right, I think I was trying to protect myself subconsciously. (Jane)

A tiny bleed. A car crash. Both fine. (Jenna)

Lots...fibroids, unexplained bleeding, fibroid under placenta, pre-term labour at 26 weeks, at 36 weeks when doctors burst the water bag cord prolapse took place. Immediate (and dramatic) emergency C-section then took place. (Cheryl)

Chapter 11

Linsey's journey

In June 2012, Linsey gave birth via elective Caesarean section to her daughter Kezia. Linsey was keen to share her experience of finding out she was expecting a baby with Down's syndrome and how it affected the rest of her pregnancy. For more information about Down's syndrome have a look at one of these websites:

www.futureofdowns.com
www.downs-syndrome.org.uk

'Down's syndrome is one of the most common genetic causes of learning disability and around 750 babies are born with the condition each year in the UK. Down's syndrome affects people of all races, religions and economic background equally.

The condition is caused by the presence of an extra copy of chromosome 21 in a baby's cells. It occurs by chance at conception and is irreversible. As yet, no one knows what causes the presence of the extra chromosome 21.

Although the chance of having a baby with Down's syndrome increases with age, babies with the syndrome are born to mothers of all ages. There is no evidence that anything done before or during pregnancy causes the syndrome.'

Source: www.nhs.co.uk

After 8 years trying to have kids with my ex-husband, you can imagine my surprise when, less than 6 months into a new and fairly casual relationship and just after my 37th birthday, I realised I was pregnant. It's not that I don't understand cause and effect; I had just assumed it would never happen to me.

As my periods had been regular as clockwork since some gynae procedures about 18 months earlier (and, let's face it, 8 years of becoming hyper aware of my cyclical monthly changes), I started feeling a strange mix of hope and desperation (in case my hope once again got dashed) within a few hours of auntie flo turning up late. I called my best friend, just because. I managed to wait 2 days before finally deciding to do a pregnancy test.

I had been working late and met my OH at the pub when I finished. On the way back to his flat he wanted to pop into Tesco for supplies and I put a test in the basket! First he knew.

We hurried back to his place with him all excited at the prospect and me trying to play it down and not get my hopes up. I peed on it, got 2 lines (although one was faint) but managed to convince myself and OH that the test was faulty and sent him to the local 24 hour garage to buy another one, but they didn't sell them.

So, next morning I bought a digital test on my way home. Peed on it and then realised that it didn't work as it was 6 months out of date. I bought 2 more on the way to work and tried again, but this time missed the stick with my pee! I was now well and truly peed out. I drank a pint of water and had a coffee and then drove to my first appointment of the day. On arrival, I disappeared into the loo, finally managed to pee on another stick and got the result 'pregnant'. I stared at it for a few minutes, fully expecting the 'not' to appear afterwards like a cruel, teenage prank, before I sent OH a text and then get game head on to deliver a 2 hour seminar on Domestic Violence.

I was ecstatic. Completely over the moon. And miserable as sin as I faced a foreseeable future of no smoking, drinking or blue cheese. I had a total and utter miserable grump on for at least a week.

Fast forward through the next 2 months which included moving in together, 3 early scans I got at Saint Thomas' hospital in London and the best Christmas EVER telling my parents they would be finally getting their first, long awaited grandchild. As 12 weeks fell on Boxing Day I had my growth scan at 13 weeks. My parents came along to the scan with me and we were all excited to see the baby, who was now identifiable as such.

My first inkling that something was wrong was when the scan went on longer than expected and the sonographer was muttering to herself and then mumbled something about having to get her boss. The crux of it was that despite opting out of the screening tests the nuchal fold (a tiny measurement taken at the back of the baby's neck) was much larger than it typically should be, indicating possible physical or chromosomal differences. After a moment of stunned silence, my Mum piped up 'oh well, we will all love it anyway', which just about summed it up. We were invited to return the next day to see a doctor to 'discuss our options'.

Return the next day I did, this time with OH instead of my parents. I was rescanned and we were essentially told we had a 1:3 chance of a chromosomal problem, of which Down's was the most likely, and a 1:5 chance of a physical problem, of which a heart condition was most likely.

Because of my age, OH and I had talked about the possibility of having a baby with Down's. One thing we had both agreed on without argument is that we would not terminate nor would we have an amniocentesis or CVS due to the risk of miscarriage. Although low, neither of us wanted any procedure that carried such a risk. We talked things through at length with the doctor and came up with an agreed plan, which basically meant we would have frequent scans to look out for physical problems, the second trimester blood test to screen for chromosome differences and possibly a late amnio at 34 weeks so we could get a pre-birth diagnosis.

The doctor seemed somewhat surprised by our decision making and we were offered an amnio at the 3 following appointments. It is only now that I know that 90% of people would have chosen to abort the baby in our situation that I understand the approach taken. I do wonder how many people who had not taken the time to investigate might have been taken down a road they might not otherwise have chosen, just because it was expected of them.

In the course of the next few weeks we had a number of results. The blood test came back 'high risk', a hole in the heart was detected and some fluid around the heart, all stacking up the odds more towards Down's. Funnily enough though, the deciding factor for me was the femur measurement coming up short! OH and I are both quite tall. In my head this, the most unreliable and vague of all the indicators, was the one that made me believe that my baby would have Down's syndrome.

It took a while to get my head around things. The most difficult time was leading up to the 20 weeks scan, when the chance of there being a problem incompatible with life was much higher than the average pregnancy. As time went on and we could start ruling stuff out it got easier and easier. For me, a live baby was what was important, not what diagnosis it may have.

I shed tears, wailed 'why me' and threatened to punch the next person who said 'the baby would be lucky to have me' (quite frankly, I was thinking about myself at this time, and I didn't feel lucky). However, on February 14th 2012 I felt real kicks for the first time. There had been flutters but this was unmistakable. From that moment on nothing else mattered. I loved my baby no matter what. I could feel it move and I had regular reminders that something was growing inside me. Kicks grew stronger and turned into alien baby rolling that looked most bizarre from the outside. As space got more limited, the hiccups increased (the baby's, not mine) and I would take great pleasure in watching the bump jerk up and down.

And so to the 34 week growth scan. We decided we did want an amnio. By this time I knew there was something different. If it wasn't Down's it was something else, and at least I knew about this particular syndrome. We had the test on the Monday, where we were also told the baby was quite big, and a consultant appointment on the Thursday. The specialist midwife came to see me at the clinic to tell me the diagnosis had been confirmed. I just felt relief that (a) I finally knew and (b) it was Down's, rather than anything else that I was ignorant about. However, that same day, I was also told that due to the baby's size and proportions, they wanted to do a Caesarean section at 37 weeks, just over 2 weeks away! THAT was the information that left me gobsmacked!

The surgery itself went pretty much according to plan. We turned up, waited around for a bit, made stupid jokes, etc, and then went in to a theatre full of strangers to whom I bared my bottom and subsequently a lot more whilst they cut the baby loose. The screams were, unexpectedly, immediate. OH announced that we had a girl. That was also unexpected as we were both convinced we were having a boy, even though we had chosen not to find out the gender at the scans. I made him check!

She was a blue baby so I had a brief cuddle and photo before she was whipped off to special care and I went to recovery. I then didn't see her for 7 hours as I had to wait for the epidural to wear off enough for me to be fit to go and see her. To be honest, she looked odd. She had a lot of retained fluid and so was really puffy. I also struggled to associate the baby in my arms with the missing bump. I don't know how she fit in there for a start. She was only in SCBU for 24 hours and by the end of the first night on my own with her I was as besotted as her dad had been from the start.

Kezia (meaning spice tree – my nickname is tree) is simply the most beautiful baby I have ever seen. I feel sorry for everyone else I know as their babies are not as cute as mine. Luckily they all seem to feel the same way.

Chapter 12

The second trimester

So, you've made it through the first trimester. You've had your 12-week scan and have an estimated due date to meet your little bundle of joy. Perhaps your sickness has subsided (perhaps it hasn't) and maybe a bump has begun to appear. During this trimester your hospital may offer a second 'anomaly' scan between weeks 18 and 20.

I found that once I hit 14 weeks I stopped feeling so tired and sick and could start eating proper food again. At our 20-week anomaly scan we also asked to find out the sex of our baby, although this is a personal choice and not all hospitals will tell you.

How did you feel during the second trimester?

Tired (still). Worse than the first trimester! (Jessica)

Great: although I had some residual nausea throughout the pregnancy I wasn't being sick. I also felt like I had a lot more energy and I loved it when the wriggling started! By this time I'd also come to terms with the surprise and shock that accom-panied finding out I was expecting and started feeling excited about the pregnancy. (Kathy)

Pretty good, all things considered. The small amount of sickness that I had went away. I got my appetite back for tea and coffee. Although my bump was increasing in size it remained quite compact, so I was still able to walk around quite easily. The only annoying symptom that I had was quite painful hip ache in the night. I tried using pillows in various positions, but it didn't really work. (Kate)

A little tired but that might be because I'm a children's nanny and had a lot of running around to do after 3 children. (Beth)

Absolutely fine, just a little bigger! I suffered with heartburn which probably started in the 2nd trimester, but nothing that Gaviscon didn't sort out.

I was peeing a lot which got rather annoying especially at night as we have a downstairs loo, but always went straight back to sleep after. I had a urine infection again which made me shattered for a week again but antibiotics cleared it up ok.

I had glucose in my urine after getting it tested to make sure the infection had cleared so was sent to hospital for a glucose tolerance test which thankfully came back negative. (Lindsay)

At around 14 weeks my feet began to swell in which I did mention to the midwifes but they said it was normal, once I reached 17 weeks I began to feel less tired and wasn't sleeping after work before my tea. I felt very proud of my growing bump and was actually pleased to buy and wear maternity clothes. I carried on with my life as I had previously done before I was pregnant. (Em)

Fine – I even started exercising again. (Natalie)

I was pretty ok but still fairly tired. I had some joint issues as the relaxin kicked in (I twisted my shoulder putting my coat on and couldn't drive for a couple of days – it's still not right now) but nothing else once the morning sickness eased. It was great being able to walk round telling everyone too. I had a 'Baby on Board' badge and loved showing it off. (Christie)

Even though I believed I was pregnant it didn't really feel real. I didn't start showing until late into the second trimester and the pregnancy didn't impact me physically. I also didn't feel him move till quite late. Even though I was excited and I had started buying for the baby, I was mainly focused on my job and the work being carried out in the house. (Zoe)

I felt quite tired and ratty in the second trimester, I couldn't get comfy at night and I was worried about scans, etc, so I wasn't in a great way. I read up on stuff every night on BabyCentre and on books I got out of the library so I was aware of all the risks associated with the different stages. I think this made me not take for granted that I was growing a baby. (Lou)

I felt better although my morning sickness went from week 11 to 16. I felt reassured by the sickness so it wasn't a problem. I was embracing my changing body and delighted that the news was public now. (Jane)

Much better, I had no more nausea. I also had more energy and felt really well. After my twenty week scan I really started to enjoy my pregnancy, as my scan confirmed no issues with our baby.
Prior to this I'd refused to buy anything for the baby as I thought it might jinx my pregnancy. Up till this point I'd struggled to be really excited as I kept thinking I would lose the baby or my baby would have some sort of birth defect. I was so relieved

when my 20-week scan was ok and everything was confirmed as normal.

I loved being able to feel my baby kick and would often stroke my tummy to get a reaction from my baby. People would comment on it and my father-in-law said my baby would be born bald as I'd be stroking all the hair off his head.

I started to find sleeping a struggle as my baby kicked a lot, more so when I was at rest such as lying in bed. He was a fidget all the time never staying still.

I was very excited to find out I was having a boy. Whilst the main thing for us was having a healthy baby. I had also wanted a little boy (a big brother for any future children) so it felt really special. (Emma)

I relaxed a little more although I was still too scared to believe that everything was going to go well. I was still very tired especially because I was a nanny and the little girl wanted carrying around all the time! (Claire)

That's when the complications began. I was put on bed rest at about 16 weeks. There were no new bad physical symptoms. The complications started with fibroids, extended to fibroid under placenta and led to eventual threatened pre-term labour at 26 weeks. (Cheryl)

The same: I was anaemic and I was bad at eating and drinking enough. I slept a lot. (Jenna)

Chapter 13

What no-one told you about being pregnant

As we've already discovered, as soon as people find out you're pregnant the advice comes rolling in. However, I was keen to find out and share the other side of pregnancy: things that came as a surprise. I was fully expecting to feel big, possibly swollen and hopefully 'blooming'. What I was less prepared for was that my leg hair stopped growing!

Perhaps you'll share some of these unexpected symptoms of pregnancy...

So many small niggly things that I guess just get forgotten about once you've given birth like the hips increasing in size, your knees and other joints feeling like they belong to someone a hundred years old. (Natalie)

Everyone tells you everything they know about being pregnant as soon as they find out! However I think what gets overlooked is that putting your feet up, taking things easy and not lifting heavy stuff doesn't prepare you for life with a new baby. (Kathy)

I couldn't believe how quickly my fitness deteriorated. It felt as if I hit 7 months and I suddenly had no stamina. Walking up a flight of stairs almost killed me! (Zoe)

All the bits apart from sickness and cravings! Especially the non-glamorous bits, like piles and constipation. (Jessica)

You stop getting a proper night's sleep a long time before the baby is born! (Kate)

You are tired all the time, people at work make no allowances for you being pregnant, you feel fat and miserable, 9 months of not partying was quite tough, everyone has an opinion on names (don't bother telling people), you fart a lot, you have an appetite that is never satisfied, you get insomnia (I had an absolute nightmare sleeping during most of my pregnancy – I was tired all the time but went to bed and ended up awake and working at 2am regularly. (Louisa)

That pelvic pain sucks big time. Also that you could get stretch marks that appear after birth. (Beth)

How great it is! Everyone is nice to you, especially strangers, and if someone is not nice (eg, takes the last seat on the train or pushes you out of the way) then everyone around usually rallies round you and stands up for you. Also, how much you pee, even in the first trimester! (Christie)

How much you'll miss sleeping on your front, and how frustrating it is not being allowed to have a Jacuzzi/sauna/hot bath when they're exactly the things you'd benefit from. (Jenna)

You wee yourself when you cough/sneeze even with a strong pelvic floor! That upset me a lot. (Lou)

Very bad gas, it's awful. Other than that I had quite a neat pregnancy! (Jane)

I have very open friends so didn't really experience anything no-one had told me about, one friend even made me watch her birth video because she said it would make me feel better... it didn't!
It was just the severity I was surprised by... everyone tells you about the tiredness but you don't realise how much it affects you. (Claire)

Four things:

(1) Stretch marks on your inner thighs – I used Bio Oil throughout the last 4 months of my pregnancy and applied it each night everywhere but never expected to get stretch marks on my inner thighs.

(2) How much and for how long you will bleed post pregnancy – I had a good idea because of my miscarriage and mentioned it to my also pregnant friend. She said she would have worried about bleeding so heavily if I hadn't mentioned it – and it didn't come up in the antenatal classes I attended.

(3) How great it feels to be pregnant – people mention tiredness, back ache, some mention the glow of being pregnant but no-one tells you how special it feels to be carrying another little person inside you that is with you 24 hours a day. Also how vulnerable it can feel to be pregnant. I've always been quite a confident person, never worried about walking home alone in the dark or falling on my bum in the ice, but when you're pregnant you're not only looking after yourself but the little person inside, so if felt like I had a commitment to my baby to keep myself safe.

(4) That you may get the equivalent of blood blisters across your body from the exertion of pushing during labour. I had them over my neck and back for a couple of days post giving birth. I remember mentioning to my friend how strange it was when I spotted them in the mirror and she had the same thing when she gave birth. (Emma)

How long it seems to last. (Cheryl)

Chapter 14

Kathy's journey

Forget the heartache of trying month after month to get pregnant: for Kathy it was the last thing on her mind. I wanted her to share this story as it shows that despite being young and unprepared, having a baby is a challenge to which anyone can rise.

One warm summer's day I was heading from my morning job to my evening job and had a little time to kill so I did something I had never done before. I went to a pharmacy and bought a pregnancy test.

I had recently finished my second year exams at university and was working three jobs through an agency to earn money over the summer. I had split up with my boyfriend of two years a few months earlier but had recently started seeing a new guy. Things were going well but something was missing – my period! I had come off the pill when I became single. It wasn't really intentional – I just hadn't quite got around to renewing my prescription. I had an appointment booked with the family planning clinic and Ollie and I had been using condoms but I was becoming increasingly aware I was late. So I ventured into the unknown and walked into the pharmacy not really thinking I could be pregnant but I just wanted to be sure. I bought a basic test kit that was on offer for a few pounds which was basically a plastic cup and a sponge on a stick. The instructions said that if I was pregnant a line would slowly develop after a few minutes. I popped the stick in the cup and immediately a very strong, dark line appeared. No doubt at all.

I didn't really know how I felt. I didn't really feel anything. It was a problem to be dealt with. After work that evening I met my boyfriend at a pub and, finding a quiet corner, I showed him the stick. He said, 'what does this mean?' I replied 'it means uh-oh'. We didn't discuss things in depth. He said he'd respect whatever decision I made. I said there was no decision to make. It would be madness to consider having a baby. I was half way through university. He was just about to graduate with no idea about what to do next. We'd been together six weeks.

I kept my appointment at the family planning clinic but rather than asking to renew my pill prescription I explained the situation and asked what my options were. I was asked to do another test – a rather more elaborate device than my sponge on a stick – which again showed a strong positive line immediately. The doctor then started to talk about options. Keep the baby. Have the baby and put it up for adoption. End the pregnancy. Due to the doctor's religious beliefs she was not prepared to give me the signature I would need to end the pregnancy. She told me to make an appointment at the hospital where I could get the signature and a date. I procrastinated about this as something was changing in me. The cold, unemotional way I had been dealing with things no longer seemed to fit. I wouldn't however allow myself to seriously consider an alternative route.

When I eventually got the appointment made and went along to the hospital, I was about ten weeks in. We met with a rather unpleasant doctor who scolded us for using condoms as they were completely inadequate (since when?) and reminded me to be more responsible in future. I was then sent for a scan during which the screen was turned away from me. The sonographer wrote a note and folded it. She gave it to me to take to the reception desk and said there was nothing for me to see in there. Of course I had a look on the way to the reception desk. It said 'single live foetus' and my mind was made up.

Reactions
There was a mixed reaction to the news. Ollie's parents and my university tutor both tried to encourage me to change my mind. My family and friends understood why I'd made the decision I had despite the time and situation being all wrong.

That first trimester was mostly spent in a state of confusion and nausea. I had quite bad morning sickness so my morning job in a canteen with all the food smells wasn't good and the nausea would persist all day. By the time I'd come to a final decision I was almost at the end of the first three months. I'd been warned that the first three months carried a relatively greater risk of miscarriage. I used to worry about that, thinking if it happened I'd have brought it on myself by considering ending the pregnancy. Not at all logical thinking – welcome to pregnancy brain!

The second trimester
The start of my second trimester began with my dating scan. This was an altogether different experience to my first scan. I watched my baby wriggle and 'cycle' on the screen. I couldn't quite believe it was real! Despite the fact there was still a lot of uncertainty about the future and how we'd get through it, Ollie and I started to feel a bit more optimistic.

My summer jobs came to an end and as soon as the agency realised I was pregnant I got dropped like a hot potato. Ollie hadn't got the degree results he had wanted to go on to do an MSc so had gone to one of our lecturers for advice and it was suggested he look into a PGCE. At the time the training package for PGCE students looking to teach maths was quite generous and meant we'd have a little income. He also got a weekend job at a retail store and persuaded his manager to give me a temporary job. I'd chosen to take a year out from university as the baby would be due in the middle of the last semester. We didn't have much money but we had enough to get by and our friends and family really rallied around to help us out. We got a 'shop soiled' pram which was actually in great condition for a really good price. We borrowed a beautiful cot and were given a lovely Moses basket. We moved into a rented house and Ollie's dad helped me turn the spare room into a nursery. My father and stepmother cleared and decorated the downstairs for us. It became a home but it still didn't feel quite real!

Although I came from a big family (only one brother but my mum was one of seven and my dad one of eight), I was one of the younger grandchildren and none of my friends had children so I had no experience of pregnancy or babies. I didn't know what to expect. I read pregnancy books avidly – 'studying' for pregnancy almost. I knew exactly what a textbook pregnancy should be but I still got caught out from time to time like when I started producing milk at six months! I had bags of energy throughout the second trimester and loved the feeling of my wriggly baby. At the second scan we chose not to find out the baby's sex. I had no preference but Ollie really wanted a boy. I picked up white, yellow and green vests and sleep-suits. We opened one out and quickly packed it away again – scared by how tiny it was! I wrote my birth plan with my midwife. Stay at home for as long as possible. Bath and gas and air only. Find out the sex ourselves. Nope – still didn't feel real.

The third trimester
My third trimester passed quickly. I still felt energetic (just as well as I couldn't drive, so I

walked everywhere). My diet wasn't great. My appetite had never quite recovered from morning sickness so I mostly lived on Diet Coke, potatoes, mushy peas and Haribo! My job came to an end and in those last couple of months I got a kidney infection and toothache which were both pretty unpleasant experiences. However they passed and I looked forward to my due date, excited about the next phase of giving birth and meeting my baby. I turned 21 and had a very sober party at a nearby restaurant. I had my hospital bag packed and waiting by the front door. Ollie would head off each morning wondering if today would be the day he'd get 'the call' to come home and take me to hospital. My due date came and went and nothing happened. Over the next two weeks I'd get the same phone calls every morning – any news? No nothing yet. My midwife started talking about induction and made an appointment. Don't worry she said, you probably won't need it. The night before my appointment I spent on my hands and knees adding the final coat of varnish on the large wooden floor downstairs. Baby had no plans to move!

Labour

The following morning Ollie drove my mother and me to the hospital and headed off to school. He had a teaching assessment as part of the PGCE course. After an hour or so waiting the doctor visited on his rounds. He examined me and declared my body wasn't ready to have the baby. I was given a pessary to get things going but was told not to expect anything to happen until after the weekend. This was Wednesday.

I played cards with my mum for a few hours. We got some lunch and read some magazines. Just after we'd eaten I started experiencing light cramps like period pains and a dull ache in my lower back. I mentioned it to my mum and she said it was probably nothing, bearing in mind what the doctor had said. Ollie turned up having had a successful assessment and my mum said goodbye. After an hour or so I was really very uncomfortable. Ollie went to get a midwife who gave me aspirin and recommended I get into a bath. She doubted I could be in labour as the pessary usually took longer to take effect. After about 30 minutes in the warm water my discomfort became unmistakable contractions rising like waves to a peak then descending. Ollie again fetched the midwife who checked me and to everyone's surprise I was 4cm and in established labour.

I was moved upstairs to the birthing suite. I got in the bath there and was given gas and air. We were left on our own. Ollie didn't know what to do. I didn't know what to do either. I started to feel quite scared. The contractions were crashing one after the other fairly relentlessly by this point and I felt like I couldn't cope. We called the midwife and I asked for an epidural. The anaesthetist came along and prepared me for the procedure. The gas and air was making me feel quite delirious. It is an intoxicating substance for a girl who has not drunk for some time! The placing of the epidural was remarkably quick and straightforward. The anaesthetist declared it was the quickest he'd ever done. Within a few minutes I was numb from the waist down and felt my sanity slowing returning as the gas and air wore off.

I was hooked up to a monitor and then we were left alone again. Ollie settled down for a sleep. I couldn't get comfortable. If I lay down the monitor belts slipped and the alarm would sound so I had to sit up. My mum had left magazines for me to read but they were out of reach and I didn't want to wake Ollie up. I had a very boring few hours. Not what I had expected at all – I thought labour would be a whirlwind of activity! As we reached the early hours of Thursday morning my labour continued to progress albeit at a slower rate than before. When I reached about 8cm a doctor came in to talk about Caesarean sections. I was surprised as it seemed to me like everything was going well.

I soon reached 10cm. I had been warned that the epidural might make it difficult for me to know when to push but I could feel each contraction bearing down. Baby took a while to come through. I watched as its head was born, one ear folded completely over, eyes tight shut, tongue out. It put me in mind of a puppy. It still didn't seem real. With one last push the midwife announced 'It's a boy', Ollie yelled 'Yes!' and gave a fist pump, baby gave a gargled cry and finally it felt real.

We stayed in the hospital for one night. I was in a room with three other mothers and their babies. All the dads spent the evening crowded around the television watching the football. I was utterly exhausted. That first night a midwife had to wake me up to feed my baby – his crying didn't wake me up! The next day as we packed up to take him home, I couldn't shake the feeling that at any moment someone would turn up and say I couldn't. There had been a mistake. I couldn't look after a baby. But of course no-one did. We went back home and got ready for the next stage of being parents. I spent the evening with my baby in my arms and couldn't believe what we'd created. I was head over heels in love.

And then...
Reality soon hit. Ollie qualified as a teacher and got a job. I still planned to go back to university to finish my final year so we looked at how we would manage with the cost of childcare as well. Tax credits had just been introduced but being a full time student didn't qualify us for help towards childcare costs so when Jack was four months old I started working at a nearby pub behind the bar and waitressing. I did enough hours for us to get a small top up.

When Jack was six months old I went back to university. My tutors had not actually expected me to return. I did 9–5 days every day using any free periods to study and complete assignments. I would drop Jack in to nursery on my way in and pick him up on my way home. Two evenings a week Ollie would come home and I would head out to work. Each weekend I worked on Saturday and Sunday. I hated spending so much time away from my baby. I would try and make all the time we had together count. Eventually my final year project and studying for my final exams started eating into my home time as well but by this time I had followed my mum's advice to implement a strict bedtime. You can't do this with a very small baby as they follow their own timetable, but after weaning it becomes possible and it worked very well for us as I could settle down for study after bedtime.

Looking back at how we coped with that year, it now looks like we had a tough time. My mum worried a lot that I had taken on too much. However it didn't feel like that at the time. Not returning to university wasn't an option I'd considered. I had to work for us to get by so it was just something that had to be done. I loved getting to know my little man, watching him grow, seeing his funny crawl, his gorgeous smile and hearing his first words. Every minute spent with him was a pleasure not a chore.

Ollie and I unfortunately split up once I'd graduated but he has always been very much involved in bringing up Jack. He has since had another child and Jack enjoys being an older brother at his dad's and an only child at home as he feels he has the best of both worlds.

However I am in a relationship now and my friends are starting families of their own and so the time feels right for me to consider having more children. There will be a significant age gap between Jack and any future siblings (at least 13 years) so his role as big brother will be different. He may not be a playmate for a young sibling but will be a good teacher, friend and role model. Or he will be once he has recovered from the shock of having to share me. Although I did enjoy my pregnancy with Jack I'm looking forward to doing things differently this time around! Planning the pregnancy, being excited by the positive test result and being financially stable. Hopefully a taste of the sleepless nights and endless nappy changes that new babies bring will ensure Jack becomes a responsible young man who does not make me a grandmother before my time too!

Chapter 15

Sex, drugs and alcohol

A tell-tale sign of pregnancy can often be the absence of alcohol consumed on a night out! Many women chose to stop drinking altogether and indeed the National Institute for Health and Clinical Excellence (NICE) advises that pregnant women should avoid alcohol in the first three months in particular, due to the risk of miscarriage. To be honest, alcohol was the last thing I wanted when I was pregnant so I cut it out altogether. There are some medicines and pills that can be taken safely but it is always best to seek advice first. The same applies for herbal and homeopathic remedies. Smoking and the use of illegal drugs pose a serious threat to your baby and should be avoided completely. For a comprehensive guide and support, please consult your doctor or health care advisor.

So, what about sex during pregnancy? For some, the very thought makes them squeamish whereas others find the hormones cause their sex drive to go into overdrive! It is perfectly safe to have sex during your pregnancy (should you feel up to it) and your baby will be none-the-wiser. In the later stages of pregnancy you may find that having an orgasm, or even just sex itself, may cause Braxton Hicks contractions, which can be uncomfortable but should not cause alarm.

Your midwife may advise against sex if you have had any heavy bleeding (due to the risk of further bleeding) or once your waters have broken (due to the risk of infection). Again please consult your doctor or midwife if you have any questions or concerns.

[*Medical information from:* www.nhs.co.uk]

Thoughts on sex, drugs and alcohol

I had been off alcohol for a year before conception because of the fertility issues we had been having so that didn't bother me at all. The sex life dwindled significantly as the fatigue levels increased and my poor husband was very supportive. (Jane)

I only had a couple of wines throughout the pregnancy in which I didn't really miss. Our sex life was pretty normal until about 30 weeks while I felt unwell and very swollen so it didn't happen that often. (Em)

I probably drank once a week or so, maybe half glass of wine, obviously no drugs and definitely no sex towards the end of the pregnancy! (Lindsay)

Sex became difficult – either due to tiredness, or later on, size. It is not a time where I felt sexy about myself, or particularly to my partner. Had already given up smoking a few months before pregnancy so that was less of an issue by then: I missed drinking, in the sense of going out with friends and having a few at the weekend, massively, as that was my weekend social life and you don't tend to get invited out to stuff like that when you aren't drinking (in my friendship circle at least). (Jessica)

Missed alcohol a lot but abstained (until the last trimester when I had a couple of glasses). Sex was fine up until about 7 months when I was so fat and tired I couldn't really be bothered. (Louisa)

I didn't miss alcohol at all until the third trimester and then I had the odd glass of wine but nothing much. Personally I don't think it's worth the risk to drink or do drugs during pregnancy, it's only 9 months of your life. Sex was fine although in the last month was too difficult due to the bump (which was annoying as I was quite horny at that point!!!) (Laura)

Not bothered really. I have had 20 years of going out and partying and to be honest having a baby would be a good excuse to stay in! (Vicki)

The nausea brought on by my partner's aroma didn't help our private life! I never really got the hormonal urges you sometimes hear about, much to his disappointment. I didn't miss drinking (or smoking) while I was pregnant as the thought of it made me queasy anyway! I had a glass of champagne at New Year and again on my 21st but apart from that I didn't bother. (Kathy)

I did miss wine (no drugs for me) but had about 8 glasses over the last 2 trimesters, which was nice. I really missed getting drunk though. I also gave up smoking the month before I conceived and that was fine for most of the pregnancy except for about weeks 20–23, where I would have ripped someone's face off to get a fag and a glass of Colombard! Sex was amazing! I loved pregnancy sex. The orgasms were so intense. We kept having sex right up until I went into hospital to be induced. (Christie)

We didn't have sex during my pregnancy until a week before I was due. Mainly because my husband thought it was a bit wrong when I had a baby inside me! Also I didn't really have the inclination. I think I would be more relaxed about it next time especially nearer the due date as it's meant to help things along!!

Alcohol I found hard to give up but only because my friends and family love it so much. I had one or two glasses at functions and major events though.

I found it hard not being able to have Lemsip when I had two bad colds though. (Lou)

I wanted sex but my husband wouldn't or didn't....very annoying. I don't drink but did miss cold medicines. I work with children so I pick colds up a lot and pregnancy made them ten times worse. I felt like death. (Beth)

None – I didn't miss anything I gave up during pregnancy – and I'm not much of a drinker now. (Emma)

Was definitely more lax on alcohol second time around – had hardly anything first time but probably a couple glasses of wine a week from about 10 weeks onwards second time. Never taken drugs! Also I had more caffeine in second pregnancy but still not much. I wasn't bothered by sex whilst pregnant apart from near the end when it was just too darn uncomfortable! (Rachel)

Sex: we tried our best.

Drugs: I tried to avoid everything, even paracetamol, until I got a chest infection and then bronchitis. I had to take something then, doctor's orders.

Alcohol: nothing, I knew if I had one drink I would want another so I didn't have any. (Natalie)

As soon as you get over not wanting to [have sex] because of fear of harming the baby you physically find it too difficult! Not having desserts with alcohol in them (my favourites), and cocktails was difficult!! (Jenna)

Had to abstain for 6 months and although I missed sex, the sacrifice was worth it. I do not tolerate the idea of drugs or alcohol during pregnancy. (Cheryl)

I did initially miss alcohol during pregnancy especially as I would go out and see friends and they would be drinking, I did look forward to having a drink after birth but realised it doesn't really fit in with breastfeeding, now after 4 months of breastfeeding I would rather carry on breastfeeding as I really love the bonding. (Claire)

Chapter 16

Love it or loathe it?

For Mel (see Chapter 8) being pregnant was torture and not an experience she is going to repeat. For the majority of my pregnancy I loved it – the bump, the kicks, the wonder of growing a new life. Towards the end, however, I was hot, tired and desperate to meet our baby. Here are some thoughts on the positives and negatives about being pregnant.

I loved being pregnant because...

I loved all the firsts...first time you hear a heartbeat, first time you feel it kick, first time you're aware you can't do your trousers up, etc! Loved the scans, especially at 20 weeks 'cos it's so obviously a proper little person inside you! (Rachel)

I'm a big show-off and loved being the centre of all that positive attention. I also loved my bumpy – no worries about looking fat! Seriously though, it really brought DH and me together and we shared a closeness beyond any we had previously had. It was truly amazing. (Christie)

I felt somehow special and precious for a short while as I was growing something amazing in me. (Lou)

I have to be honest, I didn't really love being pregnant at the time, although looking back it was amazing knowing there was a person growing inside of me, and when she started kicking it made it all the more real. (Laura)

You get to see a very nice side to most people. It wasn't an enjoyable experience for me personally, although the idea of the end product was lovely, but I did like having him to myself when he became a more concrete idea later on in the pregnancy. (Jessica)

I loved my bump and feeling my baby move and hiccup, etc! I loved how kind people were and considerate (most of the time) – that is, offering seats on the bus and moving out of my way on the pavement. People were so interested in the baby, asking to touch my bump (friends and colleagues, not strangers!). (Lindsay)

I didn't really love being pregnant. I quite liked eating (but not so much now) and was glad I had no really bad symptoms like morning sickness. (Louisa)

I loved the feeling of my baby inside me and looking forward to meeting them. (Kathy)

In the latter stages in particular, shop assistants, etc, would be really friendly and have a bit of a chat about the baby. I also loved feeling the baby's movements as it made everything feel so much more real, and it was like my little secret with the baby. (Kate)

It meant I was having a baby soon. (Cheryl)

I was growing a baby – our baby – and that was really exciting: an amazing feeling of the unknown! (Vicki)

I carried a life inside me, which is amazing. (Em)

Of the bonding; bonding with your partner over your shared expectations and hopes and bonding with your unborn child as you feel them grow and develop and imagine what they will look like and how they will be as they grow up. (Claire)

Knowing I was growing another life and feeling it move...awesome. (Beth)

I felt like I was strong and glowing. Although I was tired I felt empowered and so happy, lucky and thankful throughout. (Jane)

I had a life inside me, a bit of me and a bit of Jay who would grow to be their own person. (Natalie)

ಖಿ ಖಿ ಖಿ ಖಿ ಖಿ ಖಿ

I disliked being pregnant because...

I couldn't drink what I wanted or stay up late as tiredness ruled everything. (Lou)

I loved everything about the feeling of being pregnant. I was worried about what came afterwards. (Kathy)

I like having my own space: literally, in an internal sense and externally, in a personal sense, you don't get much of that during pregnancy. (Jessica)

Getting fat and being tired all the time. I also hated that you can't just decide when your baby is born (I am a bit obsessed with control). (Louisa)

Of the paranoia and constant worry that you would lose the baby. (Natalie)

I couldn't have sex or do anything but lay down in bed. (Cheryl)

Of not being able to get a good night's sleep for much of pregnancy due to one reason or another – feeling thirsty, aching hips, needing to get up to go to the toilet. (Kate)

I felt so ill for such a long time. (Jenna)

I had to do that stupid diabetes diet! (Christie)

First time around because I just didn't feel right and no-one seemed to be listening to me as other friends I spoke to didn't feel like I did. I was very scared and panicky sometimes, I felt I knew there was something wrong. (Em)

I felt huge and heavy for a lot of it and found it difficult to cope with all the changes to my body. I also suffered with all the embarrassing ailments of pregnancy, like piles, constipation and heartburn! (Laura)

The sickness was definitely the worst part....and stretch marks! (Claire)

Chapter 17

Shellie's journey

I approached Shellie for her story as she is a mother of two girls who are nearly eleven years apart in age. I knew that she had found it difficult having her first daughter at a young age but wanted to share the positive relationship she has with her daughters and her new husband. Here she shares the journey she took with each pregnancy and how they compared to each other.

Tell us about getting pregnant the first time...

I was 21 when I fell pregnant with my oldest daughter Lily. I had met her father Dan at work. We were good friends and ended up seeing each other on and off for 5 months. I had joined the IT company during my year out to go travelling before going to university and decided I needed to earn some money before I went. However, I ended up working my way up in the company, being promoted 3 times and by the age of 20 was running a department and a field of engineers. I was a real career woman and had no intention of settling down or starting a family at the time.

However, one afternoon at work, I collapsed and was taken to the hospital. After numerous tests and hours of waiting, I was told I was pregnant. I was in total shock as I had been on the pill since I was 15 to help with my acne. I couldn't work it out, I had had my usual regular periods, no bump, no sickness, no tiredness; and but yet here I was, 14 weeks pregnant and, being quite young, feeling really scared. My best friend called my parents for me and they came and got me. My dad didn't speak to me for 2 days and my mum just looked disappointed. It was my sister who was my rock during this time; she had had a baby with her husband a year before and was amazing. She said everything would be OK and helped me start planning for my new arrival. Dan was also really supportive at this point; he had had 3 children before and assured me everything would be fine. I wanted to make everything work for the sake of my baby and decided to give it 100%, so we got engaged and I moved out of my parents' into a flat round the corner with him.

How did you feel during your first pregnancy?

Once I had got around the idea of becoming a mother and being pregnant I started to really enjoy it and get so excited about my new arrival.

I didn't have any morning sickness and only felt tired towards the end when I was diagnosed with anaemia. I was prescribed iron supplements, changed my diet and tried drinking liquid iron from the health food shop, but my iron levels were really low so my midwife ended up having to come round my house and inject iron in the top of my bottom every day for 2 weeks to help me.

It did help and saved me being taken into hospital, so that was good! I was so lucky to see the same midwife the whole time, which was so nice as felt I had built up a nice relationship with her and felt comfortable asking her anything!

I was very lucky with weight gain too, whether this was due to my age or not, I don't know, but I did not have to buy any maternity clothes and just wore some baggier things at the very end. I religiously put Bio Oil all over my body especially my bump and again, I may just be lucky but ended up with no stretch marks either – I love that stuff! I continued to work full time, but a month before I was due to go on maternity leave I had a bit of a scare when I woke up with a lot of blood loss. I was petrified and taken into hospital and monitored.

Everything was fine but as I had been having periods throughout my pregnancy, it was difficult to say why it happened and the hospital just said it was 'one of those things' but all was OK. My work decided the job was very stressful for a heavily pregnant lady, so gave me an extra month off paid before my maternity leave. I was very lucky and enjoyed getting everything prepared and meeting other mums to be in my area. This in fact was a lifeline for me. All my friends were either finishing uni, still at uni, travelling, working, partying and going out all the time. No-one had children, so my antenatal group were so important, to make me not feel alone and to have some friends with something in common with me at that time in my life. A few of them are still some of my closest friends and I don't know what I would have done without them.

How did you prepare for labour the first time around?

I prepared for the labour by going to my classes (we had 6 back then) and buying every magazine and book going, I was a bit obsessed but just wanted everything to be perfect. I had Braxton Hicks for what seemed like weeks and thought I was going into labour many times towards the end as I had crampy-like pains, but nothing happened. I was terrified of being out and about and my waters breaking in public, so did stay in more than I usually did towards the end. Once my due date passed I was really frustrated, very hot –

being the end of August – and had had enough! I was given 2 sweeps, to no avail, and so was booked in to be induced on the Tuesday. Luckily Lily decided to make her own arrival and on Saturday morning whilst walking round my local shops to get present for someone, I felt my Braxton Hicks seemed much stronger and were coming at regular intervals.

I just knew it felt different and remember sitting in the deli where my mum worked, having some brunch, saying I was in early labour and her laughing, saying you wouldn't be here, you would know if you were. She was wrong, I really was and could time them to the second, they were so regular and felt so much stronger than the Braxton Hicks I had been having for weeks. I went home and rested in-between the contractions. I knew from my baby group friends who had already given birth that it was best to stay at home as long as possible, so just tried to keep myself busy and had bath after bath to help with pain as they got stronger. Being in warm water just made you feel so much better, it not only eased the pain but was more comfortable too!

Eventually by 10pm I felt I really couldn't be at home anymore and called the hospital and they told me to come in. I was examined and was 6cm dilated and was put in a labour room. My waters were broken for me and I had gas and air through the night. My contractions got stronger and stronger and more frequent but by the next morning, I was only 7cm and in a lot of pain. They said I was too tense and distressed and needed to relax more to help or I might get whisked off to theatre, so they gave me some pethidine to help. This really helped me and I felt I could deal with the contractions better and therefore was less tense, allowing the baby to naturally push down. By 12pm (lunchtime) I was finally 10cm and ready to push. Lily was born really quickly, just 15 mins later and weighing 7lbs 8oz. I tore slightly whilst pushing, as it happened quite quickly, and was stitched up after the placenta was delivered.

I think the early and second stages of labour were harder than the last part as they just seemed to go on forever. There is just no set time to how long each stage takes – which, being a bit of a control freak, was just so hard for me. I thought I would be pushing for ages, being a first-time mum, but she came out so quickly just after a few pushes. I was glad I had a normal delivery but was hoping for no drugs, but they said I was in too much distress at the time to continue so had to intervene.

The stitches, however, were one of the worst after effects of pregnancy. No-one tells you how much they sting when you need the toilet and no-one tells you how unbelievably swollen you are down below. I was quite shocked and remember getting the nurse to double check it was normal! Of course, it was perfectly normal, I just found it very uncomfortable to sit down, let alone try and go to the toilet!

Lily was born with noisy breathing which they put down to some fluid on the lungs. She refused to be breastfed and from early on was given formula as she was losing too much weight. I remember everyone going home and I was left in the hospital for the first time on my own with this baby and cried. I was just so scared as felt like I had forgotten all the things I had read, like how many layers to put the baby in, or how often to feed them, etc. The first night was so hard, Lily slept really well but I found it hard being surrounded by other babies who would cry and wake Lily up and vice versa. I don't think I slept a wink! However my midwife came to see me the next morning, which was a lovely touch, and by the afternoon we were discharged.

Lily continued to have noisy breathing and then soon developed a cough. She was diagnosed with croup but continued to have a constant wheeze and the cough did not seem to go away. She was admitted to hospital at least every 4–6 weeks as it got so bad and was given nebulisers and antibiotics. During this time I had gone back to work full time as I could not afford to be on the maternity pay and had been having difficulties with her father, who happened to have mental health problems which had got worse and made him a very hard person to live with. I felt Lily being poorly all the time was my fault and I was constantly crying and just about holding things together. It was only on my weekly visit to the health visitor, I broke down and realised I was not coping either. It had been a constant battle: working, going back and forth to the hospital, dealing with her father, who was either very aggressive or did not want me to be going out, and the general day-to-day tiredness of bringing up a baby had taken its toll. I felt like I could not cope anymore and was referred to the doctors, who diagnosed postnatal depression. I was given medication and had a psychiatric nurse and eventually attended group meetings every Wednesday to help. It was like a massive weight had been lifted off my shoulders and really helped me understand that it was nothing I or Lily had done wrong.

Talking to other people in similar situations or who had similar feelings and anxieties really got me through my postnatal depression. The medication also made me feel a lot less anxious and I felt I could cope better. There is quite a stigma about it but I can honestly say telling someone how I felt was the best thing that I could have done for myself, for Lily and for everyone around me. However, life just seemed to get harder, me and Dan got made redundant from the same company and then when Lily was 11 months old and again we were in hospital, she was referred to a consultant to have further tests to find out what was causing this reoccurring cough, constant wheeze and crying after feeding.

They gave her a Barium Swallow test which confirmed she had reflux. This was surprising as she never was sick with her feeds, but acid reflux can still occur inside the body without coming out. As well as this they noticed her heart did not look as it should and we were quickly referred back to the consultant to arrange an ECG and heart echo.

The next few weeks all merged into one and were a very worrying time, but the end result was that Lily was diagnosed as having a rare heart defect which was causing all her problems. The medical name was a double aortic vascular ring. It is a cardiovascular birth defect involving the formation of the aorta and the vessels. In Lily's case the trachea and oesophagus were completely encircled and compressed by a 'ring' formed by the vessels. This can cause breathing and eating problems as well of risk of choking and can be life threatening if untreated. We were referred to Brompton Hospital in London, where she would be on a list to await surgery, and we were given baby resuscitation training just in case – a lifeline in the end. The news was such a shock, but a total relief at the same time. I knew early on that something was wrong but never really seemed to have my case heard until she had been admitted so many times. If I had been older and wiser, perhaps I would have been stronger and fought sooner for her to be tested; who knows, I just was glad we were finally getting help for her. Whilst waiting for her operation, Lily stopped breathing once, the first time, she had finished her dinner, which as usual had caused her breathing to be noisier and her coughing more regular, but literally in the split of a second she had collapsed, stopped breathing and went a waxy blue colour. It was the scariest moment of my life but, without thinking, we went into auto pilot, gave her mouth-to-mouth and called for an ambulance. By the time they got there, she was back with us, but was still taken to hospital for checks.

We waited 3 months for her operation – the longest months of my life, but I know there were babies worse off than her that needed their operations first, which made me get through it. In hindsight my redundancy, although really hard, had come at the right time as everyone was too scared to look after Lily during this time either. It meant I could give her my full attention and care, which helped me with my own depression and feeling a bit 'worthless'. Lily finally had surgery when she was 15 months old in Brompton Hospital in London and spent many weeks recovering thereafter. She was amazing and coped so well for such a little person. The surgery went really well and saved her life. Despite stopping breathing for a second time after surgery, she eventually made a full recovery and apart from having to have yearly check-ups with local hospitals, she was signed off from Brompton.

Life went on as normal and apart from her scar across her back she grew into a normal active healthy little girl. Sadly her father and I split up: the stress of a new baby, a sick child, depression, redundancy, money problems – they could all be to blame, but actually, in hindsight, we did not really know each other well enough to suddenly spend the rest of our lives together, let alone raise a family. Her father turned out to have larger problems with his mental health – drinking, drugs and violence – and when someone like that refuses any help you eventually have to put your child's welfare first. It was not a happy environment for Lily; and after police involvement I no longer felt it was a safe environment for us to live in, either. I would never change falling pregnant at a young age, or what happened after; although a very hard period of my life, I had Lily to show from it – the most precious being in my life.

When did you decide you wanted to have another baby?

Lily and I lived very happily and I finally recovered from my depression, too, after a couple of years. Although I had wished for a brother or sister for her when she was little, I was quite happy living on my own surrounded by the amazing love and support of my family and friends as usual. Years and years passed by before I happened to meet up with an old boyfriend, James, when I was 29. It was love at first sight all over again and after a year and a half we moved in together and we got engaged. We talked about having children but I was concerned about the massive age gap, as Lily was then 9, but James had never had his own children and felt he might miss out. We also were concerned about whether we could afford a bigger place, whether James was too old, being 9 years older than me, and if it was fair on Lily. After a while we just could not get it out of our heads and decided we wanted to bring another child into our world. I got my coil removed in the May and fell pregnant straight away. Unfortunately, 2 months later, whilst travelling on a train to visit relatives, I had a miscarriage. I had excruciating stomach pains and bleeding and had to be taken off the train and onto hospital. It was so sad and I cried for days. Finding out you are pregnant is so exciting that having it taken away from you not long after finding out was just so gutting.

We happened to have a family holiday booked just a couple of days later which I went on and tried to take my mind off our loss, but it was very hard. I talked to a lot of people and it was so surprising just how common it was. It didn't make it any easier but it was good to talk about it rather than pretend it never happened.

Our sadness was replaced with happiness when I fell pregnant again straight away. I took the first few weeks after I found out really easy, just in case, as at the back of my mind I almost felt like I was waiting for it to happen again, it was so scary. I had some early spotting at about ten weeks and had to go in to hospital to check everything was OK. Luckily a scan showed it was but it wasn't until I was past the 12-week stage that I began to relax – and of course started telling everyone.

How did the second pregnancy compare to the first?

The pregnancy felt so different and nicer this time round, even know I knew from early on and was scared of miscarriage again, it just felt better. I think this was down to the fact that it was planned, everyone was excited rather than worried and it really helped that I was in a really stable loving relationship. I was working part time throughout my pregnancy and although I did have another child to look after she is much older than a usual sibling would be, so I didn't have to run round after a toddler or anything.

It was very exciting and, in a weird way, I felt like I was pregnant for the first time as it had been such a long time. I had morning sickness very early on until about 9 weeks and was very tired, but walking to and from work and school each day kept me active, which is so important. I put on just under 4 stone by the end of my pregnancy and had a huge bump – nothing compared to my first pregnancy, where I just put on a stone! I had sweet cravings this time round too and found myself not wanting anything unless it was sweet. I also got terribly itchy all over, the doctors said it was just my skin stretching and nothing to worry about but did give me some cream to help with the itching as it used to literally keep me awake at night sometimes. I also got very bad heartburn towards the later stage and lived on Gaviscon! Also, because I was so big, I got really bad backache and had to double up a spare duvet and sleep on it to help the pressure on my hips when I lay on my side. It sounds like I had all these terrible symptoms, but in a weird way I enjoyed them as I had not experienced them with my first and just felt so lovely being pregnant. In fact, it was such a different pregnancy compared to my first that I was convinced I was having a boy – which in the end, was not the case!

My baby was also breech for many months so I spent a lot of time cleaning floors, bouncing on my birthing ball or playing music to my belly to try and turn the baby round the right way. It worked at first, only for her to turn again and again. By the time I was overdue, I had a positioning scan which confirmed she was no longer breech, but back to back instead. This can cause a long and painful labour, but she could still turn naturally during labour so I felt better about that. I continued to stay as active and upright as possible to help, but as she was pressing up against my spine my back did suffer and hurt a lot at the end.

How did the second labour compare to the first?

I had a very laid-back approach to birth this time round. The first time round, I was very nervous and had a birth plan which I thought I would stick to, but realised you just can't plan what is going to happen and what you may need to get through it. So this time round, I just thought, I would see how I get on and not rule anything out.

Everyone had told me your second birth would be quicker and easier so I was looking forward to just popping the baby out: however, as it had been nearly 11 years by the time I was ready to give birth this was not the case.

I was six days past my due date when I started feeling really tired and had a headache, so had a bath and went to bed. I used to wake up a lot in the night needing to go to the toilet as the baby was always resting on my bladder, so got up at about 5am in the morning and after going to the toilet noticed red blood. I thought this was probably the 'show' they talk about but also felt some pain. I hadn't really been having Braxton Hicks like I had had continuously in my first pregnancy, so was not 100% sure if they were contractions or not but because of the blood loss decided to call the hospital.

They wanted me to come in to be checked as it was red blood and so I went in and was monitored. I continued to be monitored for the rest of the day. I was not in a lot of pain, but was still having some bleeding and having contractions that seemed to come and go but were not very consistent. The baby's heartbeat was also really quite sporadic so they decided to keep me on a ward as I was too early on in labour to be a delivery room. Unfortunately as this was a ward, visiting hours finished and my partner had to go home.

I found this very hard as I was on my own, in labour and not sure what was going to happen next. By the evening and after four baths to help with the pain, it seemed to be getting worse. The contractions were still very irregular, but when they did come, they were more and more painful, yet when they examined me, I was not getting any further. I could not sleep a wink on the ward and, apart from some painkillers, was not given anything else. I found myself feeling very overwhelmed and when it got to about 4am the next morning, again was having another bath in tears. The nurse decided to call James and let him come in out of hours and gave us a private room so he could be by my side rather than make him wait till 9am. It was the best present anyone could have given at that time, as I just wanted him next to me until I was ready to go to the delivery suite.

By 8:30am they felt I needed to go to the delivery suite and be given a drip to help bring the contractions on as they were still all over the place, but the pain seemed to be getting worse. My waters were broken and I was only 5cm. It did help slightly, but I also started being very sick. The doctors had advised the midwives that I was not allowed to eat or drink anything apart from water as they thought I might be in for a difficult labour; but, although the right thing to do, it made me feel even worse and like I had no energy at all!

The day went on and the pain got even worse, I tried bouncing on a birth ball, having another bath, just anything to help, but after getting nowhere with that and still having irregular contractions, the doctor was called in. The baby was still back to back which was why the labour was taking so long and I was in so much pain. They tried giving me pethidine, but did not make any difference this time, I was also still being sick and so was given an anti-sickness drip too. Hours passed and still no joy, so they then went on to give me an epidural which took 4 attempts and 2 people to finally get it in. Once it was in, I was put back on the bed and for the first time in over 24 hours, I felt like I could finally cope better with the pain on the contractions. The only thing I disliked was that my legs were so numb, I could not move them to lay on my side or anything unless James or the midwife helped me. I was monitored and the epidural was topped up when needed. The day turned into night and I finally got to the 10cm and was having urges to push all the time. However after trying to for over an hour and a half with nothing happening, the doctor was called in again. The baby's head was still too far up to be pushed out and my temperature was sky high. I had caught an infection and they decided they needed to take me down to theatre as the baby was not coming out naturally.

I found this quite scary. It all happened so quickly and I was signing a consent form going down the corridor with everyone in scrubs. I remember crying as I was very frightened of operations and really didn't want a Caesarean. They said they would try to get the baby out using instruments first and if it failed, I would have to have a Caesarean. James was amazing and reassured me everything was going to be fine. The staff were also lovely and, as they could see how distressed I was, talked to me and told me everything they were doing and said I was doing great. They had to perform an episiotomy first and then Grace was finally born via forceps at 10:59pm weighting 8lbs 7oz and placed onto my skin. I was exhausted, sick and a bit out of it, but it was the most amazing feeling: another little girl and she was just beautiful.

Grace did not latch on straight away and when in the recovery room found myself having to hand express into a tiny syringe so she had something. They gave us both some medication for the infection I had got during labour and eventually we were transferred up to a ward the next afternoon. I continued to hand express and tried to breast feed too. She would sometimes latch on, sometimes not. If she did, she did not stay on for long, so found myself feeding constantly to make sure she was getting enough. The nurses were great and tried to help me with breastfeeding no matter what time of night it was; but no matter what I did she just fussed a bit and never seemed to be getting enough. I stayed in hospital for 3 more days partly due to my infection and partly due to my struggle with breastfeeding. I felt like a failure watching all these other mums breastfeed away when I found it so hard. I also was incredibly swollen and sore from the episiotomy and just wanted to be in my own home, so was relieved when they finally allowed me to go home.

My feeding difficulties continued and I was worried about Grace not getting enough milk so just tried my best to feed and also hand expressed in the early days. Having a newborn, albeit wonderful, was harder than I remembered and I don't recall sleeping, let alone having a meal for the first week. I also had the shock of my life when over a few days, I literally thought my insides were falling out down below! My health visitor had come to check on me and I had asked her to check my stitches and look down there as it looked a bit strange and she advised me to go and see the doctor as she thought I had prolapsed! I was mortified and embarrassed and booked in to see the doctor the next day. It got twice as bad overnight but, to my relief, once the doctor took one look she said it was actually part of the placenta which had been left inside and was literally hanging out. It was soon removed and I felt human again! A cringing story I know, but something that is worth knowing about!

My feeding difficulties went on for weeks and I was struggling to feed with bottles of expressed milk and had the most incredibly sore and painful breasts, so decided to go back to the breast feeding clinic when she was 10 weeks old and see if they could suggest anything. The lady was amazing and noticed Grace's tongue didn't come out far. She thought she might be tongue-tied and referred me to the hospital. It turned out she was and had the operation to cut it the same day. This had definitely contributed to her feeding difficulties as being tongue-tied meant Grace was not able to open her mouth wide enough to latch on properly and would slip off. It all made sense, as she wanting feeding all the time as was not getting enough when latching on and so preferred the bottle as it gave her more – so much so that she soon cried and pulled away every time I tried to breast feed, so we settled on expressing and formula. This certainly did the trick and as soon as she could finally feed properly, overnight she started sleeping through the night, had better naps in the day and generally seemed a happier baby, which continued from then on.

How did the advice differ from midwives and doctors between the two pregnancies, or was it much the same?

The general advice had not changed much, but how you prepared bottles, certain foods you should avoid during pregnancy and breastfeeding information was different. We also had more classes beforehand which covered a lot more aspects of pregnancy and birth than classes today and more groups after too.

I also really appreciated having the same midwife throughout my pregnancy the first time round. She knew me inside out (!) and by the time I was due to give birth, was at the hospital at some point of my labour to encourage me. This [second] time round I saw so many different people and had fewer appointments that I almost felt I was just another pregnant woman to quickly see and move onto someone else. That was a shame.

However, what has improved greatly is technology and scans. This time round a scan would have picked up my first daughter's heart condition, whereas back then they were not as clear. It would have saved nearly a year of worrying, but that is just the way things are. We also never had the option to get 3D/4D scans back then.

Was there anything that happened the first time that you specifically made a point of keeping the same or changing the second time?

I really wanted to breastfeed my second child and was encouraged a lot more this time round than before. Although I had problems with it due to Grace's tongue-tie, she was getting breast milk which I was more aware was so important that before.

What I did keep the same was not finding out the sex of the child. I just loved having that surprise after 9 hard months and so wanted the same.

I was definitely more laid-back this time as I had learnt that if you are relaxed with your child, they pick up on this and settle better.

Another thing I did change from the first was not buying so much. You can get a bit bombarded with what to get for your baby, but they are almost literally in clothes for 5 minutes before they grow out of them and you don't need hundreds of toys and gadgets to keep them happy.

Do you think you coped with things differently because you were older/younger for each pregnancy?

I definitely coped better when I was older. I was not only more mentally prepared but also financially in a better position, so felt less stressed to deal with costs of bring a new child into the world. Saying that, I feel I was still as good a mother at both times, as you always love and look after your child the best you can, whatever age, so I guess I just felt more stable.

As for physically, I don't feel any more tired this time round bringing up a baby, but it is definitely harder to lose the weight!

How did your first daughter react to your second pregnancy?

I have an amazing relationship with my first daughter, Lily, and told her early on that I was pregnant as I was being so sick and she was worried about me. She was incredibly excited about the pregnancy and said I had made her Christmases and birthdays come all at once as she had always wanted a little brother or sister. I wanted to make her involved as possible, so she helped looking for names, helped buying things and we also got her a Big Sister baby book – the same as one parents fill in, but this is especially for sisters to write in, put a scan picture in, draw what they think they will look like etc...which then continues after the baby is born too.

I feel very lucky that she dealt with it so well as for nearly 11 years she had been an only child; although she has older half-siblings she sees from time to time, it was different to actually having a sibling live with you. She was amazing during pregnancy, helping me with shopping and chores and is an amazing big sister to Grace now too.

Having such a large age gap actually hasn't turned out that bad at all. In fact I feel they both have benefitted in a way, as Lily got a lot of one-to-one love and attention when she was little, being an only child then; and now she is at secondary school I am able to give that same one-to-one attention to Grace. It is also handy having an extra pair of hands every now and then to keep an eye on things whilst you cook dinner, or help with shopping, etc. She still plays with her younger sister, albeit on different levels, but they already have a lovely close bond which I would not change for the world. In fact, watching some of my friends who have 18 month–2 year age gaps, I think I have it a lot easier and so am happy things have worked out the way they have.

Is there anything else you would like to add?

Only that despite all the pregnancy niggles, painful labours and sleepless night, being pregnant and then giving birth to this special person you have created is the most amazing experience I have ever gone through and I feel honoured that I am able to be a mum when so many people have difficulties.

Chapter 18

The third trimester

The home stretch! These final few weeks are a chance to enjoy your bump, prepare for the labour and get as much rest as you can. Like many other women I found it hard going towards the very end: I couldn't sleep properly at night and every day walking just left me out of breath. There was a definite waddle happening when I moved and my feet were big puff-balls. Thank goodness it was summer and I could wear flip-flops...

Of course the frustration at feeling so large was ultimately outweighed by knowing that our baby was almost with us. I remember being advised to enjoy the last few baby-free weeks, which I realise now I should have done, but at the time I was impatient to meet the Little Dude.

How did you feel during the third trimester?

Great, I liked being pregnant and felt no ill effects from it at all. I had a horse which I was mucking out every day, a border collie which I was walking and felt great. I had some tiredness around 34 weeks and I was walking slower! (Vicki)

Great – I was really very fond of my bump and still felt very well and energetic. (Kathy)

Still pretty good until the last few weeks, when I suddenly found it very painful and difficult to walk – like a very painful stitch. (Kate)

Dreadful: I was extremely swollen all over and found it very hard to walk anywhere far without having a rest.

I had a few water infections and was diagnosed with carpel tunnel for which I wore splints on my arms at night time. This was extremely painful in the daytime, even writing or straightening my hair was a big task to do.

I was very worried as after reading pregnancy books I felt I was developing pre-eclampsia, after many trips to the midwifes they did not agree.

So I suppose I was very anxious throughout the last stage as I felt things were not quite right. Just before I reached 37 weeks I had very high blood pressure. (Em)

Fed up! After about 6 months I felt like I had been pregnant forever and that last trimester when very slowly. I felt huge quite early on as well so only felt like I was getting even more huge by the second! (Laura)

Fat and fed up!! (Louisa)

Tired again, still craving orange juice and my pelvis hurt to high heaven. The strange thing was, only sitting was uncomfortable; walking, standing and lying down were fine. (Beth)

Really big! The heartburn was pretty bad and the peeing was ridiculous!

Towards the end my fingers felt weird, kind of numb and a little swollen. I had taken my rings off probably at the start of the 3rd trimester which is sensible as I've heard of women that have had to have their finger rings cut off!

I was very breathless and even walking up my stairs was challenging! I never got swollen ankles though thank god, or any stretch-marks strangely! (Lindsay)

I felt fine, although I wasn't. My blood pressure was high and so rest was required, I had to give up all activities and exercise. (Natalie)

My third trimester was relatively short as Callum was born prematurely; however I continued much the same as in my second trimester.

I had a scare at 29 weeks when I suffered some bleeding, however a foetal monitor showed that my baby's heartbeat was strong and it was confirmed that I was not in labour as my cervix was not dilated.

I had a few days off work to calm myself down and I took things slightly more easily after that. (Emma)

Er...tired?? And HUGE. And not attractive in the slightest. I couldn't wait for it to be over by the end. (Jessica)

I was fine in the third trimester, a lot more settled and happy. I think feeling the baby move helped me feel reassured things were going OK. It was only when I went overdue that I became a bit of a moody monster again as I was bored and hot in the middle of July. (Lou)

I loved this bit. I had a huge tummy and it's amazing how many people smile at you (in central London!) when you're pregnant. I did develop gestational diabetes though, which was discovered at 29 weeks (after I measured big they scanned me and did a glucose tolerance test, GTT, which came back very high). That was quite scary worrying how it might affect the baby and blaming myself for bringing it on with too much junk food. But once I accepted that it was just one of those things and had been reassured that baby would be OK, I was OK with it. It did mean that I couldn't eat any refined sugar though and only limited 'good' carbs, which was hideous!

I also found that it was impossible to get a good night's sleep as I was uncomfortable and had to pee several times a night. Then there was the overwhelming excitement and nervousness about actually having the baby here and how I would cope. It was all very stressful, but in a good way. (Christie)

Eventually better and I loved being massive. I developed gestational diabetes so had the faff of blood testing and cutting out sugar. It was a nuisance, and I was upset initially. I worried about the baby's size and the birth being traumatic as a result. (Jenna)

I worked up until 36 weeks so I must have been OK! I remember napping lots and though I no longer felt sick, just very hungry for food, I could only eat little and often as I got heartburn – ugh!!

I finally relaxed and began to feel very excited. I enjoyed preparing the nursery as we had just moved house, I remember pulling tiles off the wall with a crowbar at 38 weeks pregnant!

I remember washing all his clothes ready to pack my labour bag – that really made everything seem real and I loved how small all his clothes were, I would hold the clothes up to my tummy trying to picture how big he would be! (Claire)

Very nervous as I tried to stay pregnant for as long as I could. Eventually I began throwing up everything I ate and had very bad acid reflux otherwise. I spent most night sleeping in a reclined sitting position. (Cheryl)

I felt fine in myself and continued to have no real issues relating to the pregnancy. As my due date loomed I started getting apprehensive about the labour and the arrival of our baby. If I'm honest I pushed it to the back of my mind and opted for the 'ignorance is bliss' approach. (Zoe)

So excited and I loved being pregnant. I was lucky to be fit and healthy throughout the pregnancy. I was counting down the days to finish work and although I was tired I felt better than I had done in such a long time. (Jane)

Chapter 19

Before and after

Making that decision to start a family, or starting one unplanned, brings with it the realisation that life will never be the same again. And I mean that in a good way, obviously, but it does cause reflection about things unfinished and then things to look forward to. In an ideal world I suppose I would have liked to be settled in a 'family' house but the future of holidays, Christmas, exploration and excitement far outweighs this small regret.

So: things you wanted to do before getting pregnant...(but never got around to doing).

I really did most of everything I wanted to as I was older when I got pregnant and had been married for 8 years. I have no regrets of having missed something vital that can't be made better by doing it with a baby. (Christie)

Travel, do a PhD, get a job, buy a house, be with my partner for more than five minutes! (Kathy)

I would have liked to get my MSc out the way first to make life easier! And no doubt travelled more with staying in good hotels and drinking cocktails – harder with children – as is reading books, so maybe a few more of those! (Jessica)

Finish the kitchen and nursery! (Zoe)

Do a Master's, to have moved before I got pregnant (ended up moving at 38 weeks), have had a few more holidays just as a couple, enjoyed a few more nights out, been more financially prepared. (Claire)

More exotic holidays. More nights out. drinking. (Louisa)

Go on a cruise. Finish the house. (Lindsay)

Weekend breaks around Europe, find a job relevant to my degree, buy a designer handbag. (Em)

Travel for a year out, but that plan had been shelved before planning a family.
Buy a Mulberry handbag: that'll never happen now!!
Get a bigger house in preparation: also unlikely to happen anytime soon with nursery costs, etc!
Finish paying off my loans. Get a new kitchen and bathroom. (Jane)

I'm an impulsive person so have pretty much done everything I wanted to do before getting pregnant. It would have been nice to have got married and go on a foreign honeymoon but I was at least engaged and the wedding was booked. (Beth)

Travel to Australia – hopefully we'll still do it one day (when we have much older children).
Move house – now successfully completed 2½ years later. (Emma)

Didn't have anything at the time, although in hindsight I wished we'd travelled a bit more as it's so much easier to do without kids! (Rachel)

My Master's degree in education, a European cruise, visit Egypt. (Cheryl)

I think I did everything – just! (Natalie)

ෆ ෆ ෆ ౭ ౭ ౭

Things you're looking forward to doing with your baby...

Simple things like day trips to the beach, fun fairs, snuggles in bed, going for walks and watching them grow. (Natalie)

Baking with Callum and letting him lick the spoon – we have since tried this and he wasn't interested in licking the spoon!
Jumping in puddles in Wellies – one of our favourite activities.
Teaching Callum to swim – we've been doing WaterBabies classes since Callum was 4 months old.
Curling up with Callum on the sofa watching a movie and eating popcorn – not there yet.
Duvet Sundays – lying in bed reading the papers/having breakfast in bed with Callum tucked in the middle reading a comic. (Emma)

Learning to swim.
Creative activities – drawing, making things.
Travelling.
Discovering my baby's personality.
Celebrating events like Christmas which will, I think, regain their magic with a small person in the family. (Kate)

Seeing the world through new eyes and watching a little person develop their own personality and ways. I enjoy travel with my son – he's great company. (Kathy)

I now have an excuse to go on all the rides at Disneyland.
First birthday party.
First Christmas.
Hearing my child call me Mummy.
Being able to bring a child up how I want, not how other people want. (Beth)

Holidays.
Learning about our likes and dislikes as a family. (Louisa)

Showing off the baby, going to baby groups, cuddling in bed the three of us, watching Daddy and baby together, lots of new adventures and milestones. (Em)

Holidays; reading together; cooking together; lots of cuddles; the parenting experience as a whole as a family unit. (Jessica)

Taking her to Australia to see my brother and his family.
Going skiing (eventually!).
Watching her grow and develop her different skills.
Christmas! (Laura)

Travelling, learning. (Cheryl)

Travelling when she gets older. Taking her to dancing classes like I did when I was a child. Doing Christmas for her and making it magical, making all our own traditions. Doing her hair (if she ever gets any). Teaching her to play the piano. (Christie)

Don't remember having specific things I was looking forward to, other than the general stuff of all the firsts and watching their development...First smile, laugh, sitting up, crawling, talking, walking, etc. I think it wasn't things I was looking forward to DOING as a family, rather it was just BEING a family in the normal everyday stuff. (Rachel)

Getting married with Harry as a part of the ceremony; first family holiday in Spain on Harry's birthday, swimming and on the beach; seeing Stuart and Harry bond over cars and boy toys; seeing him grow up with my best friend's baby who was born 3 weeks before; hearing him say Mummy and Daddy! (Claire)

Going to Alton Towers and Disney World. First family holiday to Centre Parcs! Trips to Pizza Hut/McDonalds for treats. Going for bike rides in the woods. (Lou)

Teaching him; seeing things through his eyes; being excited with him; relaxing with him; Christmas. (Jenna)

Chapter 20

Thoughts about labour

I suppose I thought about labour from the outset as part of the whole baby-making process. I'll admit I watched far too many TV documentaries filmed in labour wards, which increased my curiosity as to how I was going to react in that situation. I have a fairly healthy relationship with my body and thought I could trust it to know what it was doing when the time came. What did concern me was not being in control at any point and like many women I'm sure, the thought of doing a poo during labour (it happens) mortified me!

What were your thoughts about labour?

I'm a pretty squeamish person and before I seriously thought about trying to get pregnant, the labour was something that I didn't think that I would be able to handle very well. However, as soon as I got pregnant, I felt very different about it. It seemed more like one part of the pregnancy and parenthood journey, rather than the only important event. Even as my due date approached, I didn't get too scared. Even though I had a pretty good birth, I think I might be more nervous about it another time, having heard in more detail all the things that can happen during labour from other people. (Kate)

The pain and that the baby wouldn't come out of such a small area! I comforted myself by thinking that my body was designed for this and that billions of women go through it and are fine, some even giving birth on their own! (Lindsay)

My biggest fear about labour was the complete loss of all control and of the unknown. (Natalie)

I really didn't know what to expect. I feared it might be awful I suppose. However I also felt quite resigned to it being a process I had to go through and it would be OK in the end. (Kathy)

I wasn't scared and I didn't make a birthing plan either. I just decided to wing it and see what happened, after all I'd never been through it before. I'm quite a laid-back person and don't really stress or worry much. (Beth)

Drugs all the way.
(Louisa)

I spent some time on a delivery unit when doing my nursing training, and had even assisted with a couple of births, so as such I felt very well prepared, and certainly when it comes to drugs etc. pretty knowledgeable. I think it enabled me to go in with an open mind as to what would happen. (Jessica)

I was terrified but also aware that there was nothing I could do about it. The baby was in there and had to come out so there was no point worrying about it too much! (Laura)

Whilst pregnant I never thought about labour or birth as my attitude was the baby has got to come out and as long as the baby was safe I wouldn't mind, however after doing antenatal classes I began to feel nervous and really didn't like the idea of an assisted delivery. I also had a fear of pooing during labour. (Em)

I had completed a HypnoBirthing course and was actually looking forward to it! But because the baby was breech, and despite all attempts (lots of them) to move the maggot, they were all unsuccessful so I had a planned C-section. (Vicki)

First time: fear of the unknown.
Second time: fear of the known! (that is, I know this is gonna be agony and I really do not want to have to go through it again!). Also fear of it going 'wrong' again at the end, as it did first time, and needing to have intervention, specifically C-section which was more likely second time and which I really, really didn't want. (Rachel)

I was excited about labour and prepped with the HypnoBirthing course but when it came down to it I was induced so I didn't get to use any of the techniques (the drugs made the labour come on too swiftly to use them). I really was more excited than scared about it though. (Christie)

I was never really scared about giving birth or going into labour maybe because Callum was premature I never got to the stage where I thought labour was a reality. Because I was enjoying being pregnant so much I never worried about what labour would be like, even when we started antenatal classes, although to be fair we never got as far as the ones on giving birth – we did 'signs of labour' and 'post birth' classes; that is, what would it feel like to be new parents and the commitment and routine to come. (Emma)

I feared the baby having a big head, I feared him being handled too roughly, I feared him getting stuck. I was obsessed with delaying cutting the cord. (Jenna)

I was worried that it might end up in having a C-section as I knew Stuart would have to go back to work quickly and I especially didn't want forceps as I knew you would have to have a cut. (Claire)

I wished I could have experienced natural childbirth. My experience has placed a deep fear in me for another pregnancy. (Cheryl)

I was excited by the prospect of labour but scared of the pain and of tearing. I wanted to be midwife led and use the pool. I listened to my HypnoBirthing CDs and thought I could take a bit of pain. My pain threshold isn't that low so I felt/hoped I would be able to deal with it. I didn't like to listen to other people's birth stories but they seemed to share them regardless! (Jane)

I really wanted a lovely calm natural birth. I went to birthing classes to learn techniques to open up your cervix and feel relaxed. I was terrified of needing forceps at the delivery and therefore tearing/being cut. I wanted to avoid intrusions and drugs as much as possible and thought I was capable of doing that. In the end I had everything I didn't want, an epidural and forceps delivery and it was pretty horrible getting over it, but I survived. I don't think I'd be as scared next time. (Lou)

During my pregnancy I opted for 'ignorance is bliss' and didn't really give the labour and birth much thought. I didn't have a birth plan. I knew that I wanted to try with as little pain relief as possible, however, I was not adverse to having an epidural if required. It wasn't until they told me that I would have to be induced the next day that I realised that I did have some ideals. I envisaged going through the early stages in the comfort of my home with my husband. The thought of having to be induced and go through the early stages in hospital really upset me. Luckily the sweep worked. (Zoe)

Chapter 21

Birth plans

Because it was something I thought I should do, I dutifully typed out a 'birth plan' at around the 32-week mark. I tucked it in my notes and expected the midwife to ask me about it at every subsequent appointment. Needless to say, the birth plan stayed in my notes and was never referred to thereafter.

That's not to say that I think they're a waste of time – far from it. For me, it was a chance to clarify what was important during the birth, namely keeping it as drug-free as possible, preferably a water birth and to avoid a C-section unless there was a threat to the baby's or my life.

I also discussed it with my husband so that he was aware of what was important and could relay this to the midwives and hospital staff where necessary. Writing a birth plan is not a requirement before you give birth but it might help you to think about what you would like in an ideal situation and your preferences should things not go according 'to plan'.

Did your labour match your birth plan?

I didn't have a very detailed birth plan, but nothing very unexpected happened. I had said that I would quite like a water birth, but when the time came I wasn't able to, but actually I wasn't that bothered about it at the time. (Kate)

I didn't have a birth plan; I couldn't see the point as I knew I'd have no control in what happened. (Natalie)

I didn't make one but I wasn't expecting the afterbirth to cause so many problems. (Beth)

Nope. I was planning a calm, unassisted HypnoBirth and ended up being in hospital for 4 days being induced, culminating with my waters being broken and a Syntocinon drip and an epidural. (Christie)

My birth plan was open, although it did not end up the labour that I was hoping for. (Jessica)

Nope! I hoped I would go into labour naturally (I was induced two weeks after my due date); I hoped to use the bath and gas and air only (I ended up having an epidural); and we had asked to find out the sex ourselves (the midwife announced it). However, I can't complain really – it was a textbook delivery. (Kathy)

No. (Cheryl)

I didn't write one, however I did state I didn't want any drugs, only gas and air, only if medical staff felt it was necessary and I wanted to be able to move around.

As soon I arrived at the delivery suite I had to remain on the bed on my back whilst they tried to stabilise my blood pressure whilst constantly checking my baby's heartbeat with a monitor strapped around my tummy. I did have drips and other things but was very pleased I only used gas and air, which, personally, I did not feel did much for the pain as I could not feel any build up of a contraction, so I puffed on it whilst I had full on pain. (Em)

I didn't have a plan as I was afraid it wouldn't match. I just wanted to stay midwife led if possible so that meant no epidural. (Jane)

Nope. I wanted water birth at hospital but it couldn't happen either time. (Rachel)

Not really! I had planned to use relaxation and breathing techniques, TENS machine and gas and air only as pain relief, but I had to go for an epidural in the end as it had gone on for so long. It upset me at the time but then I realised it was the best thing I could have done as it meant Steve and I both got some rest. (Laura)

Hell, no. It was the opposite. The plan was natural, no epidural, active, water if possible, home birth ideally. Diabetes meant in hospital, lying on my back in bed! I had an epidural and they had to cut the cord straight away as it was round the baby's neck. I also had a ventouse. (Jenna)

Pretty much. (Claire)

Not at all! I wanted a calm water birth but I ended up with an epidural and forceps. (Lou)

No – I went into premature labour 7 weeks early at which stage I hadn't even written a birth plan, packed a hospital bag or bought half the things you're supposed to pack in a hospital bag. We'd discussed about maybe having a water birth if a birthing pool was available at the time and had a planned visit, to see the maternity ward and labour suites, booked for the Sunday of the week Callum was born – but never made it. We didn't even know how to get to the maternity ward and hadn't planned or discussed how we would get to the hospital in the event I went into labour, given Stephen can't drive and the hospital was 30 minutes away. (Emma)

Chapter 22

Labour pains...

I'll be honest: I found labour more painful than I was expecting – well, perhaps not expecting, but certainly hoping for. It was a strange pain, though, and the rumour that you forget it all once your baby is in your arms is definitely true (it was for me, anyway).

Did you find labour more painful, or less, than you expected?

I honestly didn't give the birth much thought until they told me they would have to induce me the following day. I knew it would be painful. I found the contractions manageable however and the whole labour was relatively quick. I slept through the initial contractions. Waking at 6am I was able to cope with the pain using a TENS and paracetamol. By 12pm I was at the hospital and ready to push. What I wasn't expecting was how physically exhausting and painful the pushing was – I was pushing for over 2 hours. (Zoe)

It was just as painful as I thought once my waters had broken. Before then I thought I could handle the contractions fine. (Lou)

About the same – I always knew I wanted the drugs!! (Louisa)

I've probably forgotten now, but I'd say less painful, and certainly psychologically easier than I feared it might be. In particular, when I started to push it felt like an immense relief and not particularly painful until the baby's head started to come out. (Kate)

Less painful, more traumatic. (Cheryl)

About equal – I wasn't prepared for how relentless it was. The labour started very strongly so I was expecting 'OK' phases between contractions but they felt like seconds. (Kathy)

More: although I had an abnormal reaction to the induction gel which apparently makes it much worse (so I'm told, obviously I have nothing else to judge this against!) (Jessica)

I actually thought the labour wasn't as painful as I had expected however I pushed for over two hours to get my daughter out and felt it was never gonna happen. I didn't expect to feel exhausted and didn't realise how difficult it could be. (Em)

Equally painful but a different pain to what I was expecting. (Laura)

More painful in the early stages. But given the shortness of my labour I don't really remember how painful the later stages were, at this point I was too busy concentrating on pushing. Stephen noted he had never seen me in so much pain and how horrible my screams were but I don't remember it as being that bad. (Emma)

It was a different kind of pain. It hurt like hell but it was a good kind of pain (or maybe that's because I was off my boobs on gas and air!). It was still on of the most magical and enjoyable experiences of my life. I would happily do it all again tomorrow. (Christie)

Probably equally, but it's unlike any pain you can really imagine before you've experienced it, so in that respect it was more so. (Rachel)

More difficult; because contractions were so regular and fierce and all night and I hadn't slept so became thoroughly exhausted and out of it. (Jenna)

The contractions were more painful and difficult to manage but the actual pushing which I thought would be a lot worse wasn't as bad as I'd anticipated in relation to the contractions. (Claire)

A lot less painful then I was expecting. (Natalie)

Chapter 23

The unexpected

No matter how much you read about labour, when it comes to your own experience things may not always happen how you were expecting. As I had planned a homebirth I had read many accounts of other people's homebirths, including those that were transferred in to hospital.

I felt that knowing the possibilities kept me calm and helped me adjust when the midwife did indeed need to call an ambulance.

I wasn't expecting to make so much noise during my labour but at the end of the day I couldn't help it! The following events happened unexpectedly; and you can read some of the full birth stories later on.

Did anything else happen in labour that you weren't expecting?

Yes. I was induced, but overreacted to the gel thus ending up with uterine hyper-stimulation, which was excruciating as I had no break between contractions as they didn't stop; this was also quite scary as it could potentially affect the baby. The middle bit was OK with the actual birth but I had a third degree tear at the end and consequently had to go to surgery very shortly after he was born and remember almost nothing of the first six hours of his life.

I think in retrospect that did affect our bonding initially and I'm really glad that my partner took some photos of the actual birth moment. Also – I was about a hundred times louder than I thought I would be and threw all my clothes off and didn't care in the slightest – if anyone had said that to me before I gave birth I would have thought they were mental. (Jessica)

There was a lot of throwing up after the birth which was strange because I didn't feel sick. (Natalie)

Not really, just the afterbirth bit and being blue-lighted to hospital. (Beth)

I had an epidural after 15 hours which I planned not to prior to the birth. This was because at that stage I was not progressing as the baby was back to back so I remained at 5cm dilated for hours and there was a chance he would not spin round. I was in constant pain by then, no let up between contractions at all and after being on the go for 15 hours, I was shattered. I needed the pain to stop and have a rest. The epidural was amazing! (Lindsay)

Forceps – the fact that most people I know didn't have a normal birth. I thought ventouse and forceps would be the exception but seems not!! (Louisa)

I bled a lot throughout the labour as well as being sick, which was very degrading as I couldn't help it. I had numerous doctors and professionals come into the room as towards the end myself and Eve were struggling and I did hear them say they would need to try an assisted delivery, luckily with the help of two midwives and a doctor she finally came out. (Em)

Despite everything progressing swimmingly, at one point a doctor walked in and started talking about Caesareans! I didn't get a show and my waters didn't break which were two things I'd been expecting for weeks but apparently don't always happen. (Kathy)

I wasn't expecting to push for 2 hours and still no baby and have to resort to forceps (first time). Then I wasn't expecting labour to be so long the second time. (Rachel)

I didn't get pain relief until 7cm dilated, I would have liked some earlier! (Jane)

From the point I got into the hospital, things progressed much quicker than I, and probably the midwives, expected. I gave birth without any pain relief apart from the good old TENS machine. I certainly expected to need gas and air at the very least. (Kate)

I was surprised by how much water I had, I thought it just broke once and then it was gone but my waters kept flowing through the course of the day! (Claire)

The contractions were so close together for such a long period of time! (Jenna)

Nothing other than having premature labour and post birth not being able to see Callum for nine hours (which I never expected even though he was premature). (Emma)

It was all much slower than I had anticipated. Contractions lasted 38 hours before I was eventually put on a Syntocinon drip and had my waters broken to speed things up. At this point I was exhausted so had an epidural which meant I didn't feel the pain of crowning or actually pushing the baby out! (Laura)

The contraction pain after my waters broke was amazingly strong I couldn't breathe properly. It was so over powering. The lack of energy I had afterwards shocked me as well. (Lou)

The time of dilation was interesting. I had no idea at the time if a minute or an hour had passed. That was strange. (Christie)

Emergency C-section and being wheeled into theatre with a doctor's hand inside my vagina. (Cheryl)

After pushing for just over 2 hours I was physically exhausted and just wanted the baby out. A doctor was called and I had an assisted birth using ventouse (suction cap). (Zoe)

Chapter 24

Top things to have for labour

What are the best things to have during your labour? It seems you find out either when it's happening or a couple of hours afterwards! I remember researching the best things to take, packing my bag, re-packing my bag and then not using half of it anyway. As I laboured at home I was lucky to have everything to hand. We had bought energy drinks which were great as I couldn't stomach eating anything; and some massage oil which really helped take some of the ache away from my back and legs. Here are some essential items that our Mums found when they were in labour and during their hospital stays.

Top things to have with you during labour…

Because I didn't expect to give birth not all my essentials were packed. I did have clothes for myself and babies but that was it. Second time around I had all my music sorted which was a great distraction and took energy bars which I didn't use. I would certainly take something to do because it can be a long slow process. (Em)

I didn't need anything or particularly want anything. Post labour I would have loved to have had the following if I'd had my hospital bag ready:

My dressing gown: to be cosy and comfortable
Maternity pads: the ones that the hospital supplied, as we hadn't bought anything like that, were horrible – like bricks (Emma)

Hairband – if you have long hair.
Water bottle.
Comfy loose clothing.
Fan – if it is the summer.
Someone you love with you. (Lou)

Your own paracetamols and a birth partner who will stay awake!! (Jenna)

Pillows, a cold flannel, a TENS machine, something easy to eat (for instance, a jar of peaches, jelly). (Jessica)

I took a huge bag in with me with loads of stuff including a TENS machine and I didn't really use any of it! (Lindsay)

Bible, hope, a clear head. (Cheryl)

Reading material (and make sure it is close to you). After the epidural went in my partner went to sleep and as I had the monitor belts on I couldn't lie down to also get some sleep but couldn't reach the magazines we brought either. That was a very boring few hours. I got quite warm but the fan infuriated me for some reason but a cold flannel on my forehead felt OK. (Kathy)

My amazing fiancé, birth ball, energy drinks, disposable knickers! (Claire)

My hand-held fan was brilliant. (Jane)

A TENS machine to help manage the pain at home. (Zoe)

Nothing really – I had my iPhone and drugs!! (Louisa)

TENS machine.
Partner to do back massages during contractions!
Special, nice smelling luxury bath gel for the bath afterwards as a treat. (Kate)

Straws to aid drinking.
Calming CD – I used a HypnoBirthing CD even though I wasn't actually doing HypnoBirthing, but the music and the woman's voice were really calming and the breathing techniques helped.
Flapjacks for husband/birthing partner!
Blanket from home.
Birthing ball.
Contractions app on the iPad/iPhone – really handy as my contractions went on for so long I couldn't keep track of them without this.
Comfy nightie. (Laura)

My own music and a remote control for the iPod so I could flick past a song that was annoying me. My TENS machine was also a Godsend. (Christie)

Chapter 25

Any other advice?

As you've already seen and possibly experienced, being pregnant and raising a child invites advice from all around. There is no getting away from people wanting to help, wanting to share their own experiences and hoping that in doing so they are making things easier. Along with the advice we were given, I wanted our Mums to be able to pass on their own advice. Hopefully there will be something here that you can find helps you out.

What other advice would you like to give?

Relax as much as you can in pregnancy and enjoy being pampered and looked after. (Lou)

Whilst pregnant [if you have] any concerns do go seek advice and do not give up trying if you just don't feel right because I believe a woman's intuition is very strong and in my case I was right. (Em)

Find a support network who you can talk openly and honestly to, whether this be current friends, family, support groups or online forums. I found the online group a Godsend, talking to other women at similar stages of their pregnancy made me realise how I was feeling was not unusual. This support has continued following the birth of our children and we are now planning to meet up. (Zoe)

Enjoy the experience. It is over too quickly but at least you have a whole set of new adventures to come with your new sidekick! (Kathy)

You don't necessarily need to start wearing maternity clothes that early in pregnancy. You can keep wearing your usual trousers by feeding an elastic band through the button hole and hooking the ends onto the button. This extends the life of your non-maternity trousers significantly when you wear them with a longish top over the top. (Kate)

I did pregnancy yoga during both pregnancies which was amazing and provided me with great breathing techniques throughout labour in which the midwives did comment on, or aqua natal is relaxing too. (Em)

Sleep while pregnant, it becomes an unattainable item after birth. (Cheryl)

We actually joined NCT antenatal classes as in the area we lived none of our friends had children. The classes were well worth the money as they were full of information and tips whilst the NHS ones just gave us a quick chat about everything. (Em)

One of the best things I did while pregnant was take up dog walking. It lifted my spirits no end, got me out in the fresh air and exercising. I also hugely enjoyed cross stitching for the first time. I wish I'd organised my work/office/life better and not left so much that I'd have to do once I'd had the baby. Cooking and freezing meals was a great idea and I would do more next time. Pregnancy yoga was OK, I'm not sure if I'd go again. I didn't go to any antenatal classes and only regret that because I consequently have no friends to call upon from it. (Jenna)

You feel like the medical profession revolves around you when you're pregnant and in labour, but if everything goes well that disappears immediately after birth! Be assertive, though, if you need help – particularly with establishing breast-feeding. (Kathy)

Don't be too upset if the birth doesn't go how you expected it too as long as the baby is healthy and safe to me it doesn't matter. (Em)

Breastfeeding is not only better for your baby, it is also so, so, so much easier than bottle feeding....eventually, that is. However in the early days it is painful: really painful – and no one thinks to tell you that. But it does get better. (Kathy)

Have a lot of help on standby once you have the baby. You'll be knocked for six once you get out of hospital. (Lou)

You don't need to buy everything offered at Mothercare, etc: we did and some things, for instance a small baby bath, we never used. (Em)

It is hard work being a parent and getting used to being permanently tired. You need to have lots of patience. (Louisa)

Enjoy being pregnant and being a parent, try not to let the bad days get you down –the temper tantrums and the tears – and try to remember how lucky you are to be a parent: not everyone gets the opportunity. (Emma)

Take lots of pictures. And tag them all with a date. (Kathy)

Assuming there isn't a medical reason not to, get out and about as much as you can. It can be quite dull and lonely when your partner's paternity leave is up and you've had all the visitors and mixing that with hormones and tiredness isn't going to leave you feeling great. Some fresh air, exercise and being around other people can be very refreshing. (Kathy)

It really is true that once your baby is here, even if you've been feeling sleep-deprived during pregnancy it will not compare to how tired you feel once your baby is here. I never believed it would be so. (Emma)

Enjoy your baby while she or he is small as it doesn't last long! Lots of cuddles and love. (Lou)

Parenthood is so rewarding and I am so blessed we have two gorgeous girls. It can be emotional, scary, tiring and tough but so worth it because both of you created the life and it is lovely to watch personalities and characters develop into a young person. (Em)

I just love it; through all the sleepless nights I still feel I am the luckiest person alive to have avoided IVF and all that intervention. I thank God that the surgery sorted a lot of the problems and the extra things I did helped along the way! (Jane)

Just remember that every pregnancy, labour, birth and baby is different. It doesn't help to compare or to expect your experiences to be the same as others that you may read about. It certainly helps to read about them and have lots of information on board but don't have too strict an idea in your head about how things will be: try to be flexible and open in your planning. (Laura)

If you are planning to breastfeed attend a local support group. Breast feeding for many is hard work and takes time to perfect. Talking to those in the early stages of breast feeding will give a realistic view and ideas on how to cope with potential issues. (Zoe)

Don't expect yourself to be the perfect parent: no one is, and you will be doing a great job – instinct is a wonderful thing! A lot of advice is dished out – don't worry about ignoring it and doing things how you want, this is your child and it's up to you how you raise them. If you don't feel that bond straight away, don't worry – it's not like that for everybody, sometimes it takes a little time to get to know one another, and that's fine too.

Motherhood is hard: the sleepless nights are (almost literally) a form of torture and you won't love every moment – go in with realistic expectations – but believe me when you get a sniff of that baby head, or your first smiles, it is all completely worth it. (Jessica)

Chapter 26

If I did it all again...

Having survived your nine months of pregnancy, made it through the birth and now enjoying your new arrival, a certain reflection on how you approached it all is natural. Like many I think I would probably hope to be more relaxed the second time around; not because it would be any less important, but because I would have more faith in my body, in the support around me and because I would know I could trust my instincts.

What would you do the next time around?

I would probably try and take things a little easier especially in the third trimester. I was still doing lots and I should have rested more. (Lindsay)

I would get excited a lot earlier! Being a mum is the best thing in the world but it was the fear of the unknown that affected the first trimester particularly. (Kathy)

I have had another baby and I certainly did not worry as much, as I had another child to look after, I felt blessed to have one but of course I wanted everything to be perfect. I certainly was more assertive with the midwives as I didn't want to go through the heartache of giving birth and having your baby in special care. Throughout the third trimester I did slow down a little and had afternoon naps. (Em)

I would like to eat healthier all the way through and do more swimming and yoga. Realistically I will eat just as much junk food and do even less exercise as I will be running round after the current child. (Christie)

Not eat for four!!! (Louisa)

Nothing, I would do the same including taking a good few weeks of maternity leave before my due date to have a good rest beforehand! (Kate)

I'm sure I'd be more relaxed, knowing what to expect but wouldn't do anything differently *per se* (well, except trying to do two masters modules during my first trimester as well as a full time job because that was awful). (Jessica)

Try to worry less about the little things, although I guess with a first pregnancy you are bound to worry about everything as it is all so new. (Laura)

I would get the lovely pregnancy support pillow a lot earlier on! (Natalie)

I'd try to enjoy it more. It starts to feel real when your bump starts to grow and you feel the first butterflies of your baby growing and moving, but I spent my first trimester trying not to get excited in case I had a miscarriage. (Emma)

Nothing, except maybe get more help towards the end so that I had time to rest. (Rachel)

Not a lot apart from NOT going on holiday to Italy six weeks before I was due. It was tiring and a bit stressful. Also I think I would not concentrate on the due date so much next time, it's hardly ever accurate. Every day I was pregnant after [it was predicted] it annoyed me and I had to calm myself down and keep myself busy. (Lou)

Absolutely nothing. (Beth)

I would try to relax and enjoy it more and I would try not to put on so much weight! (Claire)

I honestly don't think I would do anything differently. (Zoe)

I'm hoping not to get pregnant again. But if I do, I am praying the complications would not occur again. (Cheryl)

Get on the iron tablets straight away and the Omeprazole after 12 weeks, for the acid reflux. EAT, eat, eat! (Jenna)

Nothing. (Jane)

Chapter 27

Birth stories

At some point during the nine months there will come a time where it will dawn on you: somehow, THIS BABY HAS GOT TO COME OUT. Whether your baby is born vaginally or by Caesarean section there's no getting away from this fact.

In some twisted way I was actually looking forward to the birth. I trusted my body, I had been doing pregnancy yoga, I was fit and healthy; heck, I had run marathons: labour couldn't be that hard, could it?

I don't want to scare anyone with what follows and, as you'll read, there are some births that were straightforward and relatively pain free. There are also births that were planned as well as those that came as something of a surprise.

I'll start with my tale...

The birth of our son went partly as we'd planned. We had wanted a home water birth and it started off this way.

The day after his due date I had a stretch and sweep just to help things along. The next day, whilst walking around the zoo, I had mild contractions followed by a 'show' in the evening. By 2.30am on the Sunday morning the contractions were in full flow and we started timing them. As they were 6–7 minutes apart we phoned the delivery suite as we wanted to warn them that things were under way. 'Take some paracetamol and wait until the contractions are closer together', was the response. Same again at 4am. By 7am I knew things really were happening so they agreed to send the midwife over. I wanted to have an examination to see how far (if at all) I had dilated and was so relieved when I was pronounced 6cm and allowed to get in the birthing pool. Hooray!

I have to admit, the rest of the day passed in something of a blur. Most of the time I was in the pool (bliss) but this was causing my contractions to slow down so Ali, the midwife, encouraged me to spend an hour out of the pool and then an hour back in. During this time, I won't lie; I was in a LOT of pain. The pain was mostly in my back and down my legs which I now know is because our Little Dude was positioned 'back-to-back'. When I reached 8cm the decision was made to break my waters: we did this in our bedroom and I was given gas and air at this point too. It was the day of the Wimbledon Men's Final (!) so Dave put the TV on for the midwives (a second one had arrived, to bring the gas and air) and we stayed in the bedroom.

Having the gas and air helped, not only for the pain relief but it gave me something to concentrate on. Once my waters had been broken I was hoping it would speed things along but when meconium was found in the waters the decision was made to blue-light us to the hospital. Now, when we had decided on a home birth, it was on the agreement that should hospital be suggested I wouldn't fight it. To be honest I would have agreed to anything at this point, so off we went.

I remember keeping my eyes closed for the entire journey, mostly due to the nausea and sickness that had been plaguing me all day. In fact I did throw up again just before leaving the house...! Thankfully it was only a short journey and upon our arrival I was wheeled into my own room.

Time had flown and by this point it was about 8pm. I was examined and to my relief was given the green light to start pushing. For about an hour I pushed, moved positioned, and pushed some more but nothing was happening. I was expecting to feel this overwhelming urge to push but it never came. They strapped me up to a monitor to check the baby's heart rate and then became concerned as it was dipping when I pushed.

The next decision was made to help him out and get us into surgery. Forms were thrust in front of me to sign and I remember being very vocal in my insistence on doing this naturally. Dave got scrubbed up as we were wheeled in and they gave me a spinal anaesthetic to give me some pain relief for the forceps assistance. This was absolutely amazing – the pain in my back and legs was now gone and I think I relaxed for the first time since being in the pool back at home. Using the forceps and with an episiotomy our gorgeous son, all 10lbs 2oz of him, was born at 10.37pm. He was placed on my front for a quick cuddle then whipped away to check everything was ok. He gave a cry straight away and scored highly on the Apgar so was wrapped up and given to Daddy.

All in all it was quite a day and not exactly as I had envisioned. However, as I'm sure every parent will tell you, the most important thing was that he arrived safely. We stayed two nights in hospital so they could monitor us both closely. Due to the meconium in the waters they wanted to check nothing had been swallowed by Owen. I was thankful for being in the hospital in the end as I was able to get support with establishing breast feeding and we were shown how to bath him and do his nappy. Bringing him home was rather surreal and now, a year later, he has grown into an independent, smiley and cuddly little boy.

Natalie's Story

Despite wanting a natural birth, Natalie's baby was breech and reluctant to move. She was scheduled a Caesarean Section and thankfully it all went smoothly.

The only thing I didn't want was a C-section so obviously that's what I got. My little baby was breech and in such an awkward position it was the only safe way to deliver her. I tried an ECV, which is where a consultant tries to turn the baby. She turned a quarter way three times and three times she turned back so there was no choice, I had to have a C-section.

I had wanted a natural birth so much that at first I felt a bit cheated. I wouldn't get the surprise of when she would be born; my baby's birthday had already been set. I worried that I wouldn't feel like I'd actually given birth as there would be no labour and no pushing.

I needn't have worried about any of these things. As soon as you see that little baby everything else becomes irrelevant.

She was here safe and sound and she was mine. She knew me, she knew the sound of my voice and I knew her. Instinct kicks in and you just know things, you know what your baby needs.

The C-section itself was very straightforward and the team of surgeons and midwives I had around me were amazing. They made the experience a relaxed and exciting one. After my initial panic attack (before the surgery/birth even started) I asked to have a running commentary on what was being done to my body. It's an odd sensation as you can feel everything but there is no pain. I was told when they had hold of my baby and when they were pulling her out of me. It felt like a basketball being taken out of my stomach.

They left a lot of her cord on so Jay could still cut it and have that experience. She was then placed on me for skin-to-skin contact and Jay and I were left with our daughter while I was stitched up. I was so amazed just looking at my little girl that I was barely aware of anything else going on.

Em's Story

Em went into labour three weeks early and was monitored very closely throughout the labour due to her blood pressure. Her little girl was admitted to the neonatal unit because of her low birth weight and initial struggle to feed. After eight days the family were able to return home together.

Just before reaching 37 weeks pregnant I went for my routine midwife appointment, where it was discovered I had very high blood pressure. I was told to stay at home for the weekend as there were no available beds, not leave the house and to go and be assessed at the hospital on the Monday. I stayed at home and relaxed.

In the early hours of Sunday morning I felt dull pains around my tummy and couldn't sleep, I got up and sat in the lounge whilst my partner Andy sat up with me as was worried about me. I stood up to go to the toilet and my waters broke, I was unsure at first as I thought I had wee'd but realised I could not stop the water. I phoned the hospital and they told me to come in, because of my high blood pressure. At this stage I felt very excited that my baby was coming whilst Andy was very nervous.

We arrived at the hospital just before 4am, to be greeted by a lovely midwife on the delivery suite. The midwife went over my notes and what had happened at my midwife appointment, she asked me to lie on the bed whilst a monitor was strapped around my tummy and monitored my blood pressure; I didn't feel any pain as such, just a dull ache. After being monitored for 30 minutes it was decided I could be examined. I wasn't looking forward to this but knew it had to be done.

I was very excited to find out how many centimetres dilated I was, and was hoping for about two. Luckily for me I was 5cm.

I went to the toilet shortly afterwards and I started bleeding and having a lot of pain, Andy was with me rubbing my back and called for the midwife, she wasn't concerned over the blood loss and was very tactful as I kept being sick with the pain (unfortunately the night before I had eaten a curry), which I kept apologising for.

After checking my blood pressure again I was told I would need to stay on my back on the bed whilst me and my baby were monitored throughout the labour. The contractions increased in intensity, which made me sick, but were very infrequent, I never felt a build up so when using gas and air it didn't work throughout the contraction, I used it to bite on. A doctor was asked to come and see me and it was decided I would need a drip to regulate my contractions; after many attempts from 3 different nurses the doctor administered the drip into the cannula – when looking at my arms I had different areas bleeding from the needle marks, but I didn't care as I was away with the gas and air. I was examined again and I was 7cm after 2 hours, very pleased but getting very tired and exhausted. During some part of this time the midwife left the room to find her replacement as her shift had ended; whilst she had gone I had an urge to push, so Andy buzzed and immediately two midwives came in. The midwife told me I had a couple of hours to go, she did examine me and found I was 10cm, I was excited to know the birth would be over shortly and we could meet our baby.

I got changed into the nightie I had bought for birth and waited for the next contraction, however they started to die down, the drip was turned up but I had no build up so the midwife looked at the monitor and told me when to push. I found this very hard as I had to be lying down and just couldn't push properly.

For over 2 hours of pushing I had two midwives, a health care assistant and a doctor with me to monitor myself and my baby. Assisted delivery was discussed because of the stress on myself and baby, but luckily, after a few more pushes and being placed in a degrading position with two midwives, I gave birth to a beautiful baby girl just before 7am. When they showed me her I was over the moon. We called her Eve and I was asked how much did I think she would weigh. I knew she was small so thought about 6lbs, we were very shocked and upset to find out she was only 4lbs 12ozs. Eve was placed on my chest whilst I delivered the placenta myself which was really difficult as I had no strength left.

Whilst I was being cleaned up I had frequent visitors of medical staff, I believe now they were probably assessing Eve how well she was coping with being so small because they had told me straight away she was jaundiced.

Before I was taken to the maternity ward I phoned my parents to tell them the news, my mum cried and my dad just kept saying how excited he was to meet her. Andy tried to dress her with an outfit we had brought but everything was too big, the hospital gave us doll's clothes and premature nappies until we could get some. Eve was dressed in a tiny pink babygro, pink knitted cardigan and woolly hat to keep her warm. Whilst on the maternity ward Eve began to have difficulties as she wouldn't feed and was very lethargic; a paediatrician was called to look at her and said he would monitor her and would like me to try and feed her every two hours. Each time I tried she was not interested.

I was surrounded by other new mothers whose babies were thriving and mine wasn't which made me very emotional.

Andy went home at night time and the midwives took Eve off me so I could sleep, but that night I hardly slept with worry and at around 4am I went to find her. The midwives explained she would still not feed and her blood sugar levels were very low, it broke my heart as it was never meant to be this way. I was so tired as I kept having my blood pressure taken and I was given tablets for this.

The midwives explained the doctor would come to see me and brought Eve back to me. In the morning, all alone, a neonatal doctor came to see me and explained that Eve would be admitted to establish what was wrong; my whole world fell apart and I didn't have Andy to hold my hand. Andy was unaware of what had happened as he was bringing my parents to the hospital after a 5 hour drive from Manchester. I followed the doctor wheeling my baby along with a nurse into the neonatal unit; I wasn't prepared for what I would see and couldn't believe it was happening to me. I stood there in shock whilst they put a line into her stomach and used a cannula. A woman took me away to look at her tiny baby who was half the size of Eve to distract me, it worked for a moment and a neonatal nurse took me to the parents' room whilst I waited for the doctor.

Shortly afterwards the doctor came and explained they thought Eve had a major infection and they were treating her for that and jaundice. During this time Andy and my parents arrived onto the maternity ward full of cards, presents and balloons, to find us not there. A midwife did explain what had happened and Andy came into the neonatal unit. I was absolutely heartbroken and broke down to Andy who was being very positive and telling me she would be fine. Together we went to see Eve and hold her hand through the incubator, she now had a tube in her nose as well, I was numb and felt in a trance.

My parents, one at a time, came to meet Eve which I found heartbreaking as they were so brave saying how gorgeous she was and not mentioning her health. We left the unit to return back to the ward, everything was a blur, my parents gave me cards, balloons, presents, etc, but I didn't open them, I just couldn't. I don't think I hardly spoke to them as I was in shock. Over time my parents left and Andy and I sat cuddling saying everything would be okay.

I was moved onto a separate ward with other mums whose babies were in the neonatal unit, I was so grateful to them as they helped me get through this distressing time and be positive.

Eve spent seven days in special care and grew from strength to strength. There were times where she had a small relapse but fought back – she actually pulled out her nose tube! Andy went back to work and would come and visit in the evenings when we cared for her together, dressing her, changing nappies, bathing and feeding through the tube. I spent many hours talking to Eve in the unit and expressing milk on the milking machine and was always kept informed on her progress.

The doctors came to the conclusion after various tests that I had had pre-eclampsia which had caused Eve to stop growing. Eve came out of the incubator after 3 days in which after that we were able to hold her: I had been praying for that moment and we came home after 8 days, a family together at last.

Steve's Story

This is the account of Laura's labour as told by her husband Steve. Laura experienced a straight-forward labour but after 40 hours she decided to have an epidural to help with the pain. Her daughter was born shortly afterwards!

On Friday morning at 4.30am Laura started having contractions, but considerately of her I wasn't made aware of this until I woke up to find her on the sofa wrapped in a blanket listening to a calming CD at 7am. I got some breakfast down her and got her in the bath where she was more comfortable, with some relaxing sounds and I sat on the floor holding her hand and some cold water. I called the Central Delivery Suite (CDS) to make them aware we were likely to be popping in later, and since we had a midwife appointment anyway at 11am we went to that and after a quick assessment – which was pretty unpleasant for her involving a physical check – confirmed she was 1cm dilated. Our midwife told us to go home, stop timing the contractions (about 8mins apart at this point) and chill out for a few hours, which we did.

After lunch we went for a walk around the block, which helped speed things up quite markedly, and by about 6pm I called the CDS who basically said don't come in until contractions were 2 minutes apart. They did however make me aware they were very busy and at that time only had one bed available anyway. The problem we had was that while up and walking about her contractions were going down to 2½ minutes or less, when on the sofa or in the bath they were going back up to six minutes-plus. Laura was also quite distressed by the uncertainty that the delivery suite may close and we'd be doing a trip to another unit – heavy amounts of reassurance were involved, although of course I had no idea either.

I basically focused on keeping a 'normal' routine – eating at meal times, walking around the block, bath and lots of fluids. At this point, and throughout the entire labour, bendy straws became essential as it allowed her to drink in whatever position she was in – frequently lying on her side. By around midnight–1.30am we were both getting pretty tired and although contractions were still oscillating from 6 minutes down to nearly 2 minutes, whenever I spoke to the CDS I have to say I really got the impression that because they were busy they kept fixating on her longer rather than shorter contractions and advising us to do things to slow them down (baths) rather than speed them up (walks, which I told them did the trick).

Throughout all of this she used a TENS machine which did seem to help, if only because having the remote in her hand gave her something to focus on. I'd highly recommend getting hold of one if you can, and make sure you practice putting it on and trying it out first – we had and it still took me a while to get it set up right. Also, make sure you have some spare batteries to hand: given how dependent on it Laura became, it would have been a problem if it failed.

With bags packed and ready by the door we went to bed and I grabbed short bursts of sleep while timing contractions on an iPhone app, which was really useful to give us an idea of the trend and how many longer contractions she was having rather than shorter. By 6am, however, I had decided whatever they said we'd go in since at the least I wanted to have an idea of how far along we actually were.

Again when I called the CDS it was the same story – we're busy and you should stay at home, emphasising they'd send us home if we weren't far enough along. I got some toast (didn't go down too well) and chopped banana (much better – softer) and juice down her first.

We arrived to a 40 minutes wait until they had a room ready, along with another couple in the same situation; but once we got in a room and she was assessed and found to be 5cm, we 'definitely weren't going home'. Laura was extremely relieved about this, but by this point pretty whacked. Adrenalin was working for me!

The rest of the day was a cycle of bed, ball (they had one we used), bath and monitoring (first continual but after an hour they went down to 15 minute checks).

Her contractions became so frequent that she couldn't get any food down and had very little energy as a result. In the bath the time between them extended which we used to feed her to get energy levels back up. Lucozade Sport was very useful, although I'd suggest checking the Mum likes the flavour before packing it. Laura didn't, early on, but did later most likely as her body was craving sugar.

Pain was becoming an issue by early afternoon and eventually we decided to go for an epidural. This involved a drip in her arm first to pump saline to keep blood pressure up, and also as a route to put in more drugs if necessary. The epidural going in wasn't pleasant, not least because she was contracting and had to hold still while they did it, but once in made a huge difference, although she did find it slightly distressing being confined to the bed with tubes coming out of her. On an epidural you're not allowed food or fizzy drinks, so water and Lucozade Sport was the way forward.

Probably because after 40 hours of no sleep, etc, she was so tired, her contractions were slowing down and she was still only at 7–8cms. We decided to progress things with drugs which fairly swiftly increased contractions to around 4 every 10 minutes (they aim for 5), and shortly after (within an hour) she was getting the urge to push. After that it was all over in what felt like 5 minutes, although I worked out was probably 40 minutes.

I won't lie – Olivia was born into a nasty pile of gunk and her skin was a purple/black colour, although after a quick towel down her colour lightened pretty quickly and she was breast feeding within 30 minutes, which was pretty extraordinary to watch.

Here are a few things you may find useful.

Challenge and question everything. To Laura's amazement I remembered BRAIN – Benefits, Risks, Alternatives, Intuition and No. What the midwife suggested we basically did, but Laura hearing me questioning why each time, in that format, telling them we'd discuss it and get back to them in ten minutes, I think really made her feel they were decisions we made for the right reasons.

Back massage. The base of the spine rub was essential during contractions, particularly later on. When contractions start, spend a lot of time finding exactly where and how hard she likes it and find a point of reference on her back to work from. Later on when she couldn't speak through it, it was really frustrating when it wasn't quite right.

Drinking and bendy straws. Dehydration will slow labour down, so keep the fluids constantly coming.

Eating. A little and often from early on is a good idea, to keep energy levels up, particularly for when eating will be harder. Laura had cravings for buttered toast but found it didn't go down too well, so soft food like banana was useful.

You. Make sure you eat and drink regularly as well. I found myself getting quite dehydrated – our hospital would feed both of us at meal times and tea/water was always on offer, but take along snacks. We had flapjacks, which were perfect for me.

Short sleeves. Massaging her back when she was in the bath my arm was in the water nearly to my shoulder at times. When she was having a contraction her body sometimes contorted around and my arm just had to follow her, until I was pretty much holding myself over the bath with one hand in it!

The hospital was really warm, so dress light, but the shirt should be a fairly sturdy material – I'm surprised Laura didn't rip mine during some contractions, but it was better she tugged on the shirt than me.

Occasionally while walking around she faced me with both hands clamped pulling around my neck – which is still a bit stiff as a result. Holding my hand/arm the nails went in a few times, so try to get some material in her hand when they start building.

Padding. I spent a lot of time kneeling on the hard floor by the bath and NHS towels are basically coarse large flannels. A few towels or some other padding you don't mind getting wet could be useful.

Baby's clothes. Make sure you know where the baby clothes are packed as you'll need to hand these to the midwife to dress your firstborn. A vest and babygro are all that's required; and a hat if you have one, although luckily they supplied ours – our healthy girl was too big for the ones we'd bought!

Jessica's Story

Jessica went eleven days past her estimated due date and due to reduced movement from her baby was admitted for an induction. Unfortunately she overreacted to the gel and ended up with uterine overstimulation and no breaks in her contractions. An epidural was offered, quickly administered and the labour progressed smoothly from there.

I was admitted to the antenatal ward at 4pm on Wednesday and the midwife gave me a Propess pessary around 5pm and said that we could go off and do what we liked and I would be rechecked around midnight/1am to see if I had dilated at all. At this point I was about 1cm dilated but my cervix was still long.

I took her advice and we made a break for it and headed to McDonald's to squeeze in dinner. I started to feel a bit uncomfortable while we were there, although nothing major – just felt a bit off – so despite my reluctance to spend any time in hospital when I could be elsewhere we decided to head back and roam the hospital corridors for a bit.

I was pretty sore by 8pm-ish though, so took some paracetamol and got in the world's tiniest bath on the ward to see if it helped, but didn't really make much difference, so I thought it seemed like things might slowly be starting and hopefully wouldn't need to go for the whole 3 or 4 day induction extravaganza. We headed back to my bed around 9pm and, starting to feel proper pain at this point, sent Lance to speak to the night midwife, mainly because I was really worried that he had been told he would have to leave at 10pm and I didn't think I was going to manage on my own.

She gave me some codeine – and I think she thought I was making a massive fuss over nothing. We put the TENS machine on as well which was really helpful and reduce the pain massively straight away.

I didn't feel anything like contractions pain or what I expected it to be like but just a constant pain in my back/middle that was really sharp.
Around 9.50pm I started getting in a bit of a panic at the prospect of being on my own and feeling like I was the world's biggest wuss who was never going to cope with labour pain if this wasn't even labour.

I think around now was when I started making a proper fuss and made Lance tell the midwife if he had to leave I was going to go and sit in the car with him all night until he was allowed back, as leaning on him when I had pain – which seemed to be most of the time – was the only thing that helped. So the midwife allowed him to stay a bit longer and said she would do a trace to see if I was having any contractions but that it was too early for another vaginal exam, and that we would go from there.

After the trace machine had been on for about 15 minutes she said she was going to call the doctor and she decided to do the vaginal exam after all and remove the pessary. My cervix had only got to 2cm, at which point I decided I would never be able to cope with labour pain and got really despondent and started bawling my eyes out, whilst apologising to all the other women in the bay for making a fuss and I am sure some of the 'sounding like a cow' noises were starting to creep in at this point.

However, I finally got allowed the gas and air which was brilliant and helped me manage a bit better. The registrar came and looked at the trace and said that I had a reaction to the pessary which had caused me to go into uterine hyper-stimulation – basically, instead of starting labour off slowly, as intended, I had gone from nothing to full on in about 2 hours and the reason that I wasn't feeling contractions was that I was having almost solid contractions without a break in between instead. (She was right; she showed me the trace which showed me as having one contraction for 18 minutes straight, I think, which I am pretty sure was around the point I said I wanted to die).

Anyway, I didn't realise this at the time, but it can cause foetal distress and Christopher's heartbeat was dropping at that point so they were trying to decide whether to just get me straight into theatre for an emergency C-section or whether to try and stop the induction (which was a bit counter intuitive given that is why they admitted me) or whether to give me more induction drugs to speed everything up to get me into active labour.

I can't really remember anything else from here until they got me up to the delivery unit about an hour later or so, apart from the pain, which was the worst thing ever; the gas and air and TENS were helpful; and the doctor trying to get a drip in me getting blood everywhere. The midwife was with me one-on-one for that hour and was so nice and finally I felt like I wasn't being the world's biggest wuss about the pain. They managed to slow the contractions down a bit somehow and when I started getting a gap between them it was so much better and I could actually get on top of the breathing and have a rest in between and suddenly life felt a bit better! And although the individual contractions hurt like hell, the gas and air was enough for me to get through them and was making me feel quite good at points too.

After I got to the delivery unit about midnight, things got much better.

I threw off my clothes ASAP and didn't give a monkeys who saw me – what a relief – and carried on with the cow noises.

I was really apprehensive before labour about making a noise, but at the time I did not care in the slightest. Matching the pain level with the noise was really helpful and probably the best technique I took in with me as it gave me something else to focus on. Lance was brilliant at helping me relax and focus on each contraction – and the midwives wanted to steal him for some of the other delivery rooms too. They offered me an epidural and said it was a good idea given the hyperstimulation (guess there was still the need that I might have to go to theatre at that point anyway) and believe me I agreed pretty quickly.

The anaesthetist was fantastic and got it in in about 10 minutes and 10 minutes after that I felt back to normal again – pain free but could move my legs. It was the best feeling in the world! Labour after that was fantastic – I got some sleep, Lance got some sleep, our midwife was really lovely, the hyperstimulation calmed down (not that I really cared at that point because I couldn't feel it). I dilated at around 1cm per hour as planned, they put me on the Pitocin drip to make sure I had strong/useful contractions and carried on with nothing exciting happening for several hours! I was just feeling hot so got wiped down with a cool flannel a lot, drank water and had a couple of puking sessions but felt relaxed and could focus on the positives again and meeting our baby. So little was happening that I could feel, in fact, that I kept up to date on Facebook and read the news on my phone.

They changed over to a student midwife and her mentor around 8am and I was re-examined and 9cm at that point, 10cm around 10am, at which point they left me for another hour to make sure everything was really ready to go and then started pushing. I assumed the pushing bit was going to be really difficult but it went really smoothly, I managed to focus my breathing really well and the sleep had given me plenty of energy, I enjoyed it really as I felt like I finally had something to do.

The midwife was brilliant at guiding me, Lance was the best cheerleader, and 2 hours later at 12.57, out he came! – and just in time as otherwise they would have had to call in the doctors, which I am sure was the incentive I needed to get him out.

After the initial moment where I saw him and he was all blue and really long and looked a bit like a Smurf my memory is a bit fuzzy. Lance managed to cut the cord without any untoward incident and Christopher and I had a cuddle and a little feed. No idea what was happening at the other end and couldn't have cared less at that point, but it was decided I had to go to theatre to repair one of the tears I had, so there was a quick blur of seeing an anaesthetist and a surgeon and signing a consent form and off I went leaving Lance alone with the baby. The next 1½ hours was spent in theatre being stitched back together with the epidural topped up to a spinal anaesthetic so I didn't feel a thing. I was totally knackered and kept on falling asleep and wasn't very with it in my head to be honest.

I was totally zonked for a good couple of hours afterwards as well, but luckily my uncle and brother had come in to keep Lance company and to help with Christopher whilst I was off in theatre as it all happened really quickly.

I had a third degree tear to the back and two front tears which they stitched up, and a couple of other grazes so it looked like a bit of a war zone down there, but they were happy with the repair job and we are hoping in the long run that I won't have any problems. Five days on I didn't have much control over the wee side of things but seems like the bum side of things was OK which was a massive relief. Lots of pelvic floor exercises from here on in!

So, in summary, for anyone who hasn't given birth yet...

Things didn't go how I expected at all in terms of labour, time, pain, etc, and I ended up with a couple of complications which weren't foreseen. The first bit was honestly the worst because I was scared that I couldn't cope with the pain, but after that it was OK and I don't feel particularly traumatised by any of it, although I do hope there isn't any long term damage. It was totally worth it and I would do it all again no question. The TENS machine was fantastic, gas and air was good too and the epidural really was brilliant. I wasn't planning on having one but it was so effective I am a total convert.

And in the end, although I started out wanting a water birth at home and it felt awful having to be induced, it was fine and I can't fault the care I received from the midwives in the hospital; and staying in wasn't anywhere near as bad as I thought it was going to be; and they got me into theatre really quickly so I was glad to be in the delivery unit already.

The one other thing that really helped me was that Lance took some pictures at the giving birth moment/just after which I was not keen on at the time and vowed not to look at ever, but I didn't feel that instant bond with Christopher like some people say they do with their babies – maybe because I missed out on the first few hours, or maybe just because, but actually going back and looking at them has been really helpful and I think has helped us bond since as my brain was able to make the link between the baby inside me and Christopher which I couldn't quite get straight off.

And now I feel like he has been here forever and I love him to bits.

Beth's Story

Beth had a very straightforward birth but suffered complications once her baby girl was born. She was taken from the birthing centre to a nearby hospital as her uterus was failing to contract. The ensuing operation was successful and Beth was reunited with her daughter and husband.

After a text book pregnancy and being a week overdue my waters went just after midnight in bed. When they went it felt like someone letting the air out of a balloon – only wet. I didn't start contracting but woke my partner to take me to the birthing centre. I had to be checked as my little girl hadn't engaged the entire pregnancy and they wanted to make sure that the cord didn't prolapse.

A nice quiet, quick journey through the town and I got to the birthing unit. They listened to the baby and did some other checks. All was fine, she still hadn't engaged but I was allowed home to wait for the contractions to start.

We got back around 2am; my contractions were just beginning to start. They weren't too bad, just an ache in the front (like period pains). So I scoffed a savoury muffin, 2 paracetamols and a cup of tea.

I sent Marcus back to bed and tried to get comfy on the sofa with a hot water bottle and the news (in the vain hope it would bore me to sleep). After an hour or so I decided to have a bath. It really did help with the pains, but getting out was hard when the water went cold. I went back into the living room and ended up bent over the sofa on my knees as it was the only way I could get comfortable. The cat was a little freaked out by the small noises I was making with every contraction but he eventually went to sleep in his basket.

By about 5–6am (I wasn't clock-watching or timing the contractions) the pains were stronger and a bit more frequent so I took some more paracetamols and had another bath. This time it didn't really help. I was also starting to feel a weird pressure in my bum (I know now that this was

Violet's head engaging but at the time I had no clue). The contractions were still only at the front so I'm glad I didn't hire a TENS machine. I eventually got out of the bath and woke Marcus. I decided I was going to phone the birthing centre again as I really didn't like the bum pressure. They decided I was ready to come in, so we left again for the birth centre at 7.30am.

We seemed to get stuck behind everything on the way there: three tractors, a level crossing and a school bus.

I was moaning at Marcus to hurry up but avoid all the bumps as they set off contractions, a tall ask down country lanes.

We got to the birthing unit at 8am and they had to fetch me a wheelchair to kneel in as I got halfway down the corridor and couldn't move.

Cathy was looking after me and had filled the birthing pool up for me ready. I got comfy on my knees leaning over their couch and stayed there. Cathy got me to lie down just while they did a quick examination to see how dilated I was and to listen to the baby. I was quite surprised when she said I was ready to push! I really didn't think I was that far along. They said I could get in the pool but I was like 'nope, I'm comfy here'. I mooed my way through some big contractions, I didn't need any pain relief and Violet was born at 9.07am, little more than an hour after I turned up. We found out why she hadn't engaged until the contractions started: Violet's cord was really short. Cathy had to cut it before I could have skin-to-skin (which was nice, even if Violet poo'd on me). I had the injection to hurry the placenta along but it still took half an hour.

That's when the problems started. Cathy wanted to stitch my 2nd degree tear and realised I was having these little gushes of blood. I was stitched up but was still gushing. By this point Marcus said I was white as a sheet and phasing in and out of consciousness. Cathy and the four midwives game me some honey and orange juice to try and give me some energy and hooked me up to a bag of fluid. Marcus was holding Violet while I just apologised for making a nuisance of myself (I hate fuss). By 10am the ambulance had arrived to take me to the hospital 25 minutes away. Cathy came with me massaging my uterus to keep it contracting.

Marcus and Violet had to stay behind.

I got to the hospital and was wheeled into theatre. They were trying to find a vein to put a cannula in but the veins kept collapsing. I ended up with seven in. They explained that they were going to knock me out and try and find out why my uterus wouldn't contract. If they couldn't fix it by removing the cause they would fit a balloon catheter and if that didn't work then they would have to do a hysterectomy. Signing the paper to say OK to all of this was pretty scary. I was still apologising to people, which I now realise was pretty silly.

They gave me a little thing of medicine to drink, put my oxygen mask on and I was promptly sick over me, the mask, my hair and the anaesthetist. I was cleaned up and knocked out.

I came to in recovery. The nurses were asking lots of questions to make sure I was coming round OK. The first 'was it my first child?' 'Yes.' 'Did I want more?' 'Definitely!' It takes more than what I had been through to put me off. They explained that I had a catheter and a balloon catheter fitted. The balloon catheter was filled with saline and pressed against the uterus as it contracted to help control the bleeding.

I was so pleased that it had worked and I hadn't needed a hysterectomy.

I was then wheeled to my room to be reunited with Violet and Marcus. I was cross as Violet had been given a bottle. I know she needed it as she hadn't eaten in six hours but I had left instructions for her to be cup or syringe fed if it was needed. I still had all seven cannulas in and was hooked up to two different drips. I'd lost four litres of blood and had three transfusions. I was still on oxygen and couldn't sit up much in bed.

The midwife helped me get skin-to-skin with Violet as holding her was impossible with all the drips and wires. Violet didn't want to latch on at first so we just cuddled. She then bobbed herself over to my boob and latched on all by herself!

I found it really hard not being able to just go and pick Violet up, she had to be brought to me (I was bed-bound for three days), but Marcus had to change all the nappies. My favourite quote from him when doing this was, 'OMG it's like treacle!'

I had checks every hour for two days and then the on the third day they were every four hours. I didn't get any sleep so when they finally took the balloon catheter out and let me shower (I still had sick in my hair) I was so pleased but I felt like a zombie. At this point they moved me to postnatal at 11.30pm and I felt abandoned. Nobody told me anything, Marcus had been sent home, I still had a catheter fitted so wasn't able to get out of bed. I had to keep buzzing for nurses to give me my nappy stuff 'cos I couldn't get it, then try and change a nappy on my knees semi-prone in bed. Breast feeding was going well but I couldn't get Violet back into her fish tank without waking her up so she ended up sleeping on my chest, meaning I got another night of no sleep. They took the catheter out at 6am. They were going to discharge me but decided it might be best if I went back to the birthing centre for some rest and emotional support. I'm so glad I did, it gave me two more days of recovery, and I was still pretty tired for around a week afterwards but wouldn't change anything for the world.

The reason I bled so much was that a tiny piece of placenta had stayed behind and was stopping the uterus from contracting.

I didn't want to go to the hospital but I'm glad the NHS is there when it's needed. The high dependency delivery team were wonderful, as were the team at the birthing unit.

There is only one thing that still upsets me about my experience and that is I know next time I will be classed as high risk and will have to attend the hospital. The birthing centre was so lovely and it will be forever denied to me.

Louisa's Story

Louisa used her TENS machine to help with the pain in early labour. Upon reaching the hospital she continued to progress well and it wasn't until the very end that she needed some help with forceps to deliver her baby boy.

Having had very little in the way of pain or problems I started to lose my plug on Tuesday/Wednesday and then on Wednesday night at about 11pm I was having dull period pains which started every 10–15 minutes. I didn't think too much of it as so many people talk of pains coming and going. By about midnight I packed Mat off to sleep in the spare room and popped my TENS machine on.

The pains gradually got worse and at about 3.30am I ran a bath and got in – that helped with the pain. Eventually Mat told me to call the hospital, at about 5am, as the contractions were every 5–6 mins (average from when I started, on iPhone app, so actually closer).

The hospital told me to hang fire at home until I was contracting every 2–3 mins.

The pain was excruciating by this point – I got out the bath and washed my hair in the shower and then dried it (took ages between contractions). I finished packing my bag and we headed to hospital – this was 7am. I made it down my 3 flights of stairs fine and had a contraction as I stepped outside.

It was pretty painful getting to the hospital and I had to stop lots from the car park to reception. I got checked out at triage and was 5cm dilated – this was the biggest relief as I was petrified I would be sent home as I don't think I would have made it back up the stairs!

We got sent to the labour suite and had some diamorphine – I couldn't get on with the gas and air as I was starting to panic a bit.

The midwife asked how many paracetamol I had taken and I was mid contraction and stuck up 2 fingers and she thought I was giving her the V's!

I moved to an epidural at about 9am and that was fabulous. It all went well after that until Jude decided to turn around the wrong way (he had been the right way the whole flipping pregnancy) and then his heart rate dropped and my temperature went high so they wheeled me into theatre and I had the forceps and a small episiotomy. I don't really remember much apart from all the theatre staff introducing themselves to me and me saying I wouldn't remember their names and also insisting that I didn't want a C-section (I thought the consent form was the same for each and I was panicking they would just do a section).

The next thing I recall was little Jude arriving: he was whisked away and Mat went with him; that was terrifying as I didn't know if he was okay – they told me he was but I was so worried. After all that I don't remember much else. It was a good experience, despite the ending and now I can't imagine my life without Jude.

Kate's Story

Kate used a TENS machine throughout her labour to help with the contractions. She was concerned about the lack of movement from her baby so went to the hospital for monitoring. Thankfully everything was fine and Kate returned home. Her labour was straightforward thereafter.

Unlike most people, I didn't want my baby to arrive by her due date. My Mum was due to visit to celebrate a 'significant' birthday with us 5 days after my due date. I obviously have a very obedient baby, as she held on until the night after we'd celebrated my Mum's birthday, when I started to get contractions about 2am. They started about 20 minutes apart and it was rather difficult to sleep, partly due to the sensation of the contractions and partly due to the excitement that things had kicked off. In retrospect I wish that I had tried a bit harder to sleep as I didn't appreciate that I would still be at home the following night, with much more intense contractions, and hardly getting any sleep at all.

The following day was kind of odd. The contractions were fairly manageable, and still about 10 minutes apart. To begin with I just went around my usual business, including a trip to the supermarket, which felt a bit surreal. I was amazed by how normal I felt between contractions. As the day went on, the contractions got closer together and more intense and I put on the TENS machine which was to accompany me throughout labour. I'm not actually sure whether it actually had any effect physically, but psychologically it made me feel more in control of the contractions.

During the following night I don't think I really slept at all. In the middle of the night I noticed some bright red blood in my pants. I'd read that this was potentially something of concern, so I 'phoned up the hospital, and they said it was probably just a 'show', but that I could go in to get checked out, which I did. They strapped me up to various monitoring machines, and eventually said that all looked fine.

The midwife gave me some quite useful advice. She told me to try to let the contractions wash over me, rather than trying to fight them. This helped me to manage them much better when we got home. The following day, the contractions were getting quite strong and ever closer together.

My boyfriend had a contractions app to measure the length and frequency of contractions. Every time I had one I would shout 'go' and then 'stop', from the other side of the flat! He got quite into it as I think that it gave him something to do.

I also got him to give me a back massage during each contraction which really helped me as well.

By the afternoon I was pretty worn out and in quite a lot of pain. I phoned the hospital a number of times – firstly because I was worrying about my baby not moving. I was told to eat some ice cream, which did the trick. Then later on, I phoned to try to go into hospital as I was really in quite a lot of pain. I was told that I was not yet ready and to have a bath. I came off the phone and burst into tears. However, the bath really did help me. By this time it was about 6 in the evening. All my family were still around by this point. My Mum kept saying that I should think about going to hospital, but I protested 'I can still talk during contractions. I'm not ready yet'. My Mum made me some scrambled egg on toast, which felt like the last supper, and shortly afterwards my boyfriend and I headed off to the hospital.

Even by this point I got the feeling that they didn't really want me to go in and was told that I would need to go back home if my labour wasn't far enough advanced.

When we arrived, we were fairly quickly shown to a room and had a repeat of all the monitoring that had been done the previous night. By 21.45 they concluded that I could stay and that I was 7–8 cm dilated. That was a huge relief. However, they then said that they would return in four hours to see how I was getting on. That was more disappointing. Four hours seemed like a very long time. Shortly afterwards I got the urge to push. I didn't say anything, but somehow the midwife could tell, and she said, 'You need to hold on. You're not ready yet'. I spent a few minutes trying to resist, and that was probably the worst part of the labour psychologically, as I just didn't feel that I was going to be able to resist much longer. The midwife said 'I'll just check anyway' and then 'Oh, I can see your baby's head! You can push now'. That was just a huge relief, and once I had stopped resisting I didn't feel any pain. It was, just as people had said to me, like doing an enormous poo!

At this point I felt totally focussed and just did exactly as the midwives said, pushing as hard as I could. I knew that the more efficiently I pushed the sooner it would all be over. Up until now I still didn't have any pain relief apart from the TENS machine. I did have the gas and air next to me, but forgot it was there. I quickly got to the point where the head was ready to come out. I remember being impressed by my boyfriend. He's fairly squeamish, but was looking at everything happening. I think he was just so amazed that he couldn't help but look. In a couple more pushes (and somewhat more pain at this point) the head and then body came out at 23.16, only an hour and a half since the midwives had agreed that I could stay. My baby was plopped on top of me. I didn't feel this immediate surge of love which people talk about (that came more progressively over the following days) but more complete relief that it was all over. After tea and toast I had the best bath of my whole life.

Zoe's Story

Zoe's labour progressed more quickly than she had expected, once she was in hospital. She used the TENS machine for pain relief and her son was born with the help of a ventouse (vacuum extractor).

I was due to be induced due to low fluids and high placenta; however a sweep initiated the contractions. I was very fortunate and slept through the initial contractions, waking at 6am when they started to get stronger. I used a TENS machine and paracetamol to manage the pain. By 10am my contractions were long and frequent enough that I felt I could no longer manage at home and wanted to be in hospital. My mum-in-law drove us to the hospital. Who knows what other car drivers thought as I was lent over the back seat moaning with every contraction!

Once we arrived at the hospital I had a short walk from the car to the delivery ward. I waited for a contraction to finish before I made a dash for it. I was too slow and had a contraction whilst leaning over the hospital reception desk! When examined I was only 3cm dilated, not in full labour; however, they didn't send me home. After approximately half an hour I was sure that I felt like pushing – the midwife was adamant that I could not have fully dilated in half an hour and to keep breathing through the contractions. Half an hour later and I realised I was pushing; again the midwife was insistent that I could not have dilated fully but I must have said something right as she re-examined and concluded that I was ready to push.

I was finally given gas and air; however, I found it hurt my throat and at some point threw it away (in hindsight I should've kept it!).

I tried all sorts of positions, one which resulted in me biting my husband's hand, but I couldn't push the baby out.

After over 2 hours of pushing I wanted the baby out. Even though the baby's head was slightly turned and the heart rate had dropped slightly they wanted me to keep on pushing. I was having none of it and just kept saying that I wanted a doctor and I wanted the baby out. Suddenly the room was full of people and a doctor used a ventouse to help deliver my son in one push. He was immediately placed on my chest.

Christie's Story

Christie had been diagnosed with gestational diabetes and was controlling her condition through diet rather than medication.

Gestational diabetes affects between 2 and 5 out of every 100 pregnant women in the UK. It increases the risk of the baby being large for its gestational age and therefore an induction is sometimes necessary. Christie was induced at 39 weeks.

I arrived at the ward on Thursday morning and was examined. As my cervix was slightly soft but in no way open I was given the pessary and told I would be checked 24 hours later. I had very mild period-type cramps for the next 12 hours or so. Unfortunately as it came to time for the pessary to be removed and me to move on to the next stage they closed the delivery unit upstairs and so all inductions were put on hold. I asked to be examined anyway (for my own peace of mind) and was 1cm dilated. They did a little sweep but nothing much happened. I then had to wait until 7:30pm on Saturday night to get my next set of prostaglandin (gel). This did absolutely nothing and as I had to be seen by a doctor before I could have more gel I had to wait until the next morning to be checked again. On a side note, during all this time I was expressing every 4 hours including at least once overnight each night and so I did not get great sleep.

The nurse woke me at 6am on Sunday morning and said I was still 1cm dilated but thought they might be able to break my waters. The doctor, however, disagreed and gave me a double dose of gel. Again, nothing seemed to happen. About 2pm I broke down and started sobbing. Almost everyone in my ward had been and gone (some beds multiple times) and I felt like it was never going to be my turn. This must have had an effect as an hour and a half later I was taken up to the delivery unit. They examined me again and I was still only 1cm dilated but at 4:30pm with the aid of gas and air (best thing ever btw!) they managed to break my waters. Despite contractions starting immediately they were in a hurry and started me on the oxytocin drip after an hour. I lasted about 1½ hours on my TENS machine, then moved up to gas and air once the drip kicked in. My contractions would not become regular (ranging from every 2–3 minutes to double and triple continuous ones) so they kept upping the drip. About 7:45pm I started screaming for an epidural and made rather prolific use of the F-word.

The anaesthetist came in and by 8:30pm I was weaning off the gas and air and starting to chill out a bit, albeit with about four extra holes in my back where the anaesthetist couldn't get the epidural in. During the epidural there had been a shift change and our new midwife was amazing. From there on out the whole process was like a perfect dream. I had no pain (except for needing a bit of a top up on the epidural) but I did have sensation so I could feel the changes happening to my body. We kept the lights dimmed; everything was very calm and peaceful. At 11:15pm the MW examined me. He was very careful to explain that I might not have progressed and warn us of the possible consequences but said he would hope for 5cm. However, when he looked I was fully dilated and Juan had a peek at the top of baby's head (extra surprise there that she had a full head of hair!). The MW said he would wait for an hour before starting to push to let baby come down a bit more on her own and at 12:15 we started pushing.

Sixteen minutes and five contractions later she was here and placed straight on my tummy (the cord was too short to get her any higher).

The MW let the cord stop pulsing for a minute or so then Juan cut the cord. She was put on my chest for skin-to-skin and a feed whilst the MW stitched me up (two first degree tears and some grazing – nine stitches, all on the outside). Then Juan had an hour of skin-to-skin whilst I rested (no chance of sleep – too excited!) and by 5:30am we were back on the ward and Juan was sent home.

The first few hours with a baby and no sleep were terrifying, particularly since I couldn't get out of bed to pick her up because of the catheter, but by the time Juan came back at 2pm I had the catheter out I was getting the hang of it.

All in all, it wasn't the labour I expected (or particularly wanted) but I don't feel I wasted my time with the HypnoBirthing. I used a lot of the breathing techniques through the various stages of labour and also during the induction process (for instance, before internal exams). It also took me a little while to get my head round it but now I feel quite proud of how far I got through the labour before needing stronger pain relief.

Emma's Story

Emma had not planned on giving birth before Christmas but her little boy decided to make an appearance seven weeks early. He was born naturally and spent three weeks in the SCBU before being allowed home.

I went into labour seven weeks early. I finished work as normal (I still had three weeks to go before maternity leave as I planned to finish at the Christmas break), went home, ate tea and went to bed with no idea that I would go into labour. I woke up at 2am with what felt like period pains. It went through my head that it might be labour pains – it felt different to the Braxton Hicks contractions I had experienced. I timed how far apart the pains (contractions) felt and when they were five minutes apart I woke Stephen up. He told me to go back to sleep as it was very unlikely I was in labour. The pains (contractions) did not subside and seemed to get closer together (about every three minutes). I got up to go the bathroom at about 3.30am and realised I was bleeding.

I called the maternity ward and they told me to come in so that I could be checked over. With Stephen's help I set about packing a bag with what I had available (we hadn't bought anything for the baby but had been given some second-hand clothes from a friend at work, so packed some of these along with a change of clothes for me, nightwear, towels, toiletries): I had none of the normal maternity items such as maternity pads, breast pads, disposable knickers, etc.

I decided I would drive myself but then the pain was too much. I rang the maternity ward and they told me I would need to ring a taxi as an ambulance would take at least an hour to get to me. We rang a taxi which came shortly but felt like an eternity. I panicked as I was sure when they realised I was in labour they would refuse to take me. I laid a towel down on their back seat in case my waters broke and remained quiet.

The taxi driver broke pretty much all speed limits and stated, 'I've done many things in my life but delivering a baby in the back of this taxi isn't going to be one of them'. We got to the hospital just after 5am.

A midwife took me into one of the labour suites and asked me to get onto the bed so she could examine me. At the time I was having a contraction and in a lot of pain so I asked her to wait which got a poor reaction. Once on the bed it was discovered I was fully dilated and baby was on his way. Everything then seemed to happen at once: another midwife and three doctors were called, one doctor for me, two doctors for Callum on arrival. The doctor broke my waters and I was encouraged to start pushing.

A midwife gave me gas and air to ease the pain and Stephen gave me sips of water between puffs. This was soon given up as the doctor wanted me to concentrate on pushing and I felt the need to grit my teeth which I couldn't do with the gas and air pump in my mouth.

After about 30 minutes I was given an episiotomy to help aid Callum's birth. The doctor noted Callum was starting to get distressed as he had moved into the birthing canal but I was still struggling to push him out so I put everything I had into pushing as I was determined that I wouldn't lose him from lack of trying. A few pushes later and Callum was born (a star gazer). He was placed on my chest for about 15 seconds and I just had enough time to look at him before they cut the cord and passed him to the two doctors. He did cry out at birth which gave me hope that despite being early everything would be alright.

Callum was born, weighing 4lbs 2oz, at 6.29am.

Because Callum was early they needed to take him to SCBU: Stephen asked me what he wanted me to do and I told him to go with Callum as he was the small baby and needed him more than I did. I agreed to have the injection to help pass the afterbirth and was given a pessary to numb any pain prior to my stitches (which were pain free).

I was then left lying on the hospital bed, legs still in stirrups, for about an hour. I had no idea whether it was OK for me to get down from the bed and everyone had disappeared (as it turns out due to shift change). A midwife popped her head into the room to discover me and said I could get up and have a shower, at which point Stephen turned up – told me all was going well, Callum was in intensive care in SCBU but doing fine and he had come to check on me. Stephen helped me shower and we rang family, friends and work to tell them we had had the baby, much to everyone's surprise.

I then had to wait an excruciating nine hours till 3.30pm before either of us was able to see Callum again. Another premature baby had been born, weighing 1lb 9oz at 26 weeks, and as this baby was being worked on we were unable to go into intensive care.

We tried to console ourselves with the fact that at least it wasn't our baby that was having problems but it didn't make the time pass any quicker (and it felt terrible that someone else was going through something so horrible). We asked regularly about being able to see Callum.

When we eventually made it to SCBU I cried a lot, more from the relief of finally seeing my baby properly then because he was in an incubator. We weren't able to hold him until Day 3 but we were able to hold his hand inside the incubator. He lay there, so tiny (but not as little as some of the other babies), with his mask on (he had jaundice and needed the special lights) and all his tubes and monitors and looked so vulnerable.

When I held him for the first time it felt so right and I never wanted to put him down – only being allowed cuddles initially for an hour was physically painful and I think this is why when he eventually did come home I didn't want to put him down and would just snuggle with him for hours (this lasted till he was 14 months and Stephen started making me put Callum to bed awake).

SCBU was an experience (and not unpleasant): the staff were amazing, always positive. You could visit 24 hours a day. I would sit for the best part of the day on a rocking chair next to Callum's incubator, and then crib, until Stephen came to join me in the evenings, just watching him.

The SCBU staff taught us how to hold him, change him, dress him, bathe him; and also baby CPR. I had lots of support around expressing and breast feeding but I never quite got the hang of it. From this point of view we had much more support than a first-time mum who leaves hospital the day, or day after, their baby is born with no knowledge or experience of what to expect.

Callum moved from Intensive Care into Room 4 then Room 3: we never quite made it to the 'Pre Going Home' Room as the SCBU was so full.

We followed all the advice we were given and only took Callum out of the incubator for the periods the staff recommended. Parents could do their own thing, but I believed in following their advice. We got Callum home earlier than if we had cuddled him all day long rather than letting the incubator do its job and get him well and fit to come home – whilst all I wanted to do was hold him, just seeing him lying there was the hardest thing.

Stephen was determined we would get Callum home for Christmas and on the 20th December they let us bed in (SCBU has suites where you can stay with your baby) and you stay for a few nights before they let you come home. You're left to fend entirely for yourself but you have the SCBU staff on hand if you need them.

We bedded in for three nights and it was then determined that we could go home.

On the 23rd December three weeks after Callum was born we took him home for the first time.

We were really lucky as the hospital say that when your baby is premature they aim to have you home by your due date (mine was the 20th January). So that was us: a new family, home in time for Christmas. My labour experience wasn't the best but it definitely wasn't the worst: it was relatively short and free of any major issues and at the end of it all, although somewhat later than planned, we got to take home our amazing baby boy Callum. My only wish for next time is to have a full-term baby.

Jenna's Story

Jenna's labour progressed fairly quickly and despite not planning on having an epidural she felt much more in control once it took effect. Her son was born with the cord around his neck but thankfully was healthy and happy.

I had twinges for a couple of nights but nothing major; then, having completed working on the house late afternoon on Monday and cracking on stripping wallpaper, etc, that night, and doing more on site on the Tuesday, including lots of project-managing, my waters broke while I was sitting on a deckchair in the garden waiting for my mom to come back for me. I was at the house, alone with the chimney sweep who I stood talking to about my waters breaking for 30 minutes with my legs crossed. I was surprised they popped – so I heard it pop! and they were warm: I don't know why I was surprised.

I went home and when I phoned the delivery suite they said to come in to be checked they had actually gone! I showered and washed my hair, then very calmly checked my hospital bag list, not too OCD I'm proud to say. DH was SO excited to hear my waters had gone! I was examined and was already 3cm. The exam kicked off contractions. So I was up all night with contractions every four minutes, terribly painful, wasn't offered paracetamol – and I didn't think to ask for any. I was told try to sleep, DH slept between contractions and through some, and I'm only now realising how pissed off I am that he didn't take it more seriously and support me in a more awake fashion!

The lady looking after us – this was in the induction suite, as they'd induce after 24 hours if we hadn't had him by then – said I wouldn't be in second stage until I had bright yellow show, what a crock – it never came.

They finally gave me some pain meds and I vomited them up. Checked again and was at 6cm so they sent me to the delivery suite as I'd decided I wanted an epidural as gas and air wasn't enough to dull the contractions. They were long and full on all night. I had a contraction while changing beds with no gas and air that was awful. Suffered through loads more before the epidural went in. As soon as it kicked in I was a different woman, I actually could engage my surroundings and DH and mom: so, so glad I made that decision as I was able to be present in the moment, having just been in and out of consciousness.

Labour slowed so they hooked me up to a drip to speed things up. The baby's heart rate was monitored throughout and started to dip. I had to lie on my side and have oxygen. Eventually when it was time to push I felt like I was doing a crap job but also could feel the progress and they said I did great. I could have pushed forever, but they were concerned about his heart rate. It was decided I needed a ventouse and an episiotomy when they saw the cord wrapped round his neck twice. I felt his head and thought he felt like a hairy monkey.

Cue tears, which stopped me pushing, so I pulled myself together. Out he (Seb) came and they struggled cutting the cord, but put him onto my chest and I blew on his face for his first breath, a lovely moment! Whisked off and Daddy trimmed the cord. He was returned to me for a feed. They took 50 mins stitching me up.

We spent two days on the ward where I managed to put on his first nappy backwards, put a milk bib on him which the MW removed with disdain! Had a few meltdown crying fits over not being able to breastfeed, Lord knows what else. Seb slept through all the other babies crying. I had an angel of an NCT volunteer stay with me an hour after end of her shift to reassure me I was latching him on right. I couldn't wait to get home on the Friday. Seb had to go through so many heel pricks until they had three consecutive pre-feed glucose levels they were happy with. I was so confused and getting conflicting instructions from the many MWs it took so many attempts. I had to refuse him feeds when he was hungry to get the right results and he just wailed; it was awful, so heartbreaking. Then his physical exam took ages, more screaming as they couldn't find his leg pulses.

We were very happy to get home!

Cheryl's Story

Cheryl had been put on bed rest due to unexplained bleeding and fibroids under her placenta. At 26 weeks she went into early labour but managed to stay pregnant for another ten weeks. Her labour ended up being rather dramatic but her son was born healthy and happy.

I had been having pains for about three weeks and had dilated to 3cm. I had previously been admitted for early labour at 26 weeks, which had been about 10 weeks earlier. On Friday 15th June the pain was really bad. I had a bloody show at 3am [8am GMT] and kept waiting for another sign. Eventually, more because of Anthony's panic, we went to the hospital in the early afternoon. I still had not progressed but the baby's heartbeat was causing some concern so they warded me.

On Monday morning, I had dilated to 4cm and the doctor did a membrane sweep and again I was put on the baby heart monitor. My contractions were frequent but still irregular. The nurse assured me that the baby's heart reading was fine. Fast forward to 4:45pm: I was still dilated to 4cm and told I had a long wait. At 4:50pm another doctor came in and said that I needed to be examined; I told her I had just been. She said to come with her. We met up with one of my clinic doctors and he told me they were going to induce labour immediately because he did not like the baby's heart reading. He was going to rupture my membrane and then carry me down to labour and delivery. As I was walking away he decided that he would rupture the membrane while we were in Labour and Delivery since I had already had an enema.

Within five minutes I was on my way down and Anthony caught up with us. I told him to run some errands, including keeping a doctor's appointment set months before because it would be a while. I got down to L and D and two interns were in the room. I changed into my labour gown and did whatever little odds and ends needed to be covered. The doctor invited one of the interns to rupture the membrane. She tried but failed so the doctor did it himself.

At 5:23pm he invited the intern to examine me internally and locate the head. She said she could feel it, but was feeling a squishy thing.

Everyone in the room froze, so I knew something was wrong.

The doctor literally pushed her aside and examined me himself. He called for some tools and they opened up my fadge. Apparently, it was the cord. It had prolapsed, meaning that it was preceding the baby for entry. The baby had to be delivered ASAP to survive. I was put on all fours with my head lowered to the table and the doctor's hand in my fadge preventing progress of the baby. I was wheeled into theatre and while the doctor's hand stayed where it was everyone else scrubbed up. As soon as they were ready, his hand was removed and I was put under within minutes.

My baby was born at 5:44pm. I woke at about 7:20pm in severe pain and because of my asthma I had to come to before they could administer one of the pain killers. I did not care; I started demanding to see my baby and caused quite a ruckus until my regular doctor assured me that he was fine. His Apgar was 9. It took me 2 hours to finally have him with me in recovery.

Jane's Story

Jane's labour didn't progress as quickly as she had hoped initially. With the help of a student midwife and a variety of pain-relief methods her son was born naturally.

I woke up in the morning at 2am with pains. I got up and went downstairs, didn't say anything to my husband. The pains progressed but eased on walking. I started using the TENS at 5am and decided to lie down at 7am and the pains eased so I knew I was in latent labour. I then got up at 9am and they started to come quickly then. I went for a walk in the park and the contractions came on so quickly I struggled to get home.

Three contractions in ten minutes, so it was time to phone the hospital.

They told me to go in so I made my way there. I was examined at 4pm and that was awful because I was 3cm, not in established labour, I was so disappointed but I couldn't go home because I was already struggling with the pain. They agreed for me to stay, thank goodness. I couldn't have any pain relief because I wasn't the magic 4cm dilated, so carried on with the contractions which were so strong and sore. I had a lovely student midwife looking after me and I bartered and haggled with her to get into the pool. So after a few hours of TENS and swearing as my main pain relief I got into the pool.

Unfortunately it didn't help with the pain but it did help me relax when there was a break between contractions. It escalated again and I think a combination of shouting about my human rights and begging for them to examine me earlier than planned I managed to get the midwife student to ask for me. They agreed to examine me at 7pm and I was 7cm dilated.

Immediately they gave me the gas and air, it was great, but I was still begging for pethidine, general anaesthetic, anything, but I stuck with the gas and air. I was fully dilated about and hour later so started the pushing. This went on for an hour and twenty minutes. Just as I was about to give up they said that the baby's heartbeat was dropping a little and I needed to push him out. So I managed to get him out in the next three pushes.

I had to have stitches, which were unpleasant, but I sang the whole way through them at the top of my voice, through the gas and air, mostly the Proclaimers and Dolly Parton!

So, in short, I screamed and roared and sang my way through but I managed to stay midwife led and survived the whole experience. The midwives were amazing, especially the student who looked after me!

Fran's Story

Fran's twins had been monitored closely towards the end of her pregnancy and when it was discovered that one of the boys was breech and the other transverse a C-section was considered the safest option for delivery. Fran was not expecting to go into labour a month early and in the end an emergency C-section was performed.

Both boys were delivered safely and after a short time in the Special Care Baby Unit came home.

I awoke as for a normal day, made DH a cuppa, fed the dogs and opened the door for them. DH went off to work and I went back to sleep as I hadn't slept well in the nights for months.

Woke back up (9.45am) to a stabbing pain in my back as if I needed to have a poo, so I rolled out of bed and went to the loo. One very loose poo later I felt an overwhelming urge to be sick – and I was – whilst a horrible ripping pain tore through my belly like the cramps you get to poo, and it was like food poisoning.

Except there was no food to come, up just loads of yellow bile; and vomiting whilst heavily pregnant is no fun!

So when it felt like I was empty, I was so sore I ran the bath and jumped in, and just remember seeing my bump make some weird ass shapes! I was in the bath for must've been an hour and thought there's no way I could make it to a hospital with the pain I was in, so I rang the MW and I guess listening to the way I was speaking was enough to say 'come on in'.

I 911'd DH at 12.30ish to come home, as he walked through the front door! He'd come home for lunch. He helped me outta the bath and then realised he had to run back to work. I got dressed while he did this whilst carrying my bathroom bin with me to vomit into.

Everything from there's a bit blurry: I remember getting to the hospital, DH running in to find a wheelchair and having a massive contraction in the car, then this poor woman trying to push me in the wheelchair, then a man taking over, all the while my eyes are closed and panting with my bucket on my lap and my notes in my hand. We got to the labour ward, they took one look and sent me to delivery.

Into the suite where I met the best MW I could've hoped for. Between them they stripped me into a gown, gas and air into my hand and the registrar came to scan the boys to see what they were doing.

The contractions were so bad now that I pushed down on the bottom of the bed and broke it – *oooops*. The registrar was quite happy to wait a while to see what happened; if everything stopped then we would go home or if everything worsened to go with an emergency C-section.

I had an internal and the cervix had begun to efface and was 1cm dilated but with T1 being breech vaginal birth was never an option. Ninety minutes later of sucking like a bitch on the gas and air, I was re-examined and found to be fully effaced and 4cms dilated, the registrar looked at the MWs and said something like 'Go, go, go' (slight exaggeration) followed by an NHS bikini shave, prep for surgery, husband in scrubs and into theatre.

Twin 1 was born at 4.29pm feet first, followed by his not-so-little brother at 4.30pm. I was too busy vomiting to cry. Twin 2 came to me first while Twin 1 was whisked off to SCBU with breathing difficulties and I wasn't to see him until later that night, briefly, and not to hold until much later the next day.

I was brought onto the ward at about 7pm that night with T2 having had a little suckle on the boobie and after a lot of vomiting.

Unfortunately through the night his blood glucose levels were showing low and he was taken to SCBU with his brother, where 24 hours later they were both doing great.

Liz's Story

Liz and her husband planned a home water birth. Halfway through her labour Liz was convinced she needed more pain relief but in the end she managed a natural birth with only gas and air.

I will try to keep this short, but I do believe that I had an AMAZING labour and was so lucky that everything went according to plan.

Our due date was June 2nd but as I had not even felt Braxton Hicks I felt certain we were going to be two weeks late and was convinced nothing was going to happen for at least another week. We went for drinks with friends at Hawley Lake Boat House and apart from feeling rough (as usual for me) all was fine. I was determined to get the labour going and had planned an evening of hot curry, wine, pineapple and hot sex!

We got home and I jumped in the shower while Scott started to cook the curry for dinner. I was sat on the kitchen stool in my towel when I suddenly felt something trickle down my leg. I jumped up in embarrassment that I might have actually just wet myself! I ran to the loo and Scott followed asking if I was okay.

We both through that maybe I had just had a little 'tiddle' and he continued to mock me for it.

After a minute I decided I was not in fact weeing but that this was my waters breaking! We rang the labour ward and as my midwife was due to see us in the morning we were told to sit tight and try to get some rest. I was so excited I found it really hard to sleep.

My contractions started at about 4am and felt like really strong period pains. I remember getting up to go to the loo and then not being able to get back to sleep for the contractions and the excitement.

In the morning I rang my parents as they had borrowed the pump for the birth pool for their paddling pool! They came round to drop off the pump and helped Scott to blow up the pool and see how we were getting on. My contractions were every 5–10 minutes. We had spoken to the hospital and our midwife and had been told that unless I was in 'active' labour by 7pm I would be going into hospital to be induced. To bring the labour on faster, I devoured an entire pineapple and bounced on the exercise ball like a loon! I really regretted the pineapple when I was being sick later in the afternoon...

By 3pm my midwife had come back for a second visit and I was only 2–3cm, which was very disappointing as I was no longer 'having fun'! She told me to rest and gave me some positions to try to relieve the pain of the contractions. By 7pm I was in so much pain that Scott didn't want to come near me. I kept shouting that I wanted to go to hospital and wanted the drugs for the pain. All the way through our pregnancy I had said I wanted water and gas and air and nothing else. I felt really strongly about not wanting any of the drugs for the pain. Scott, knowing I would regret going to hospital, put me off and rang the labour ward. All the labour ward did was ring our midwife who said she'd be with us by 8pm. I nearly cried down the phone to her as I just didn't know what to do with myself by this stage. Scott refilled the birth pool for the second time and we decided I should get in to help with the pain. We had been trying to put off me getting in the pool as it is said to slow down labour and we were desperate to not go to hospital and be induced.

My midwife arrived at 8pm and I was trying to relax in the birthing pool. I waddled out of the pool between contractions and remember stating that I was worried I was being a wuss!

My midwife quite rightly said if I was only 2–3cm then, yes, I was! – but I could have been 8cm. To our amazement I was indeed 8cm and our midwife called for Scott to get the gas and air. I became a much more pleasant person once I had this. The next two hours are still a bit of a blur of contractions and gas and air, all my inhibitions seemed to leave me with labour. I am usually a person who hates seeing myself naked, let alone others seeing me naked.

But when our second midwife turned up, there I was, naked in the pool with my legs spread wide. I remember going through two contractions before I politely turned round and introduced myself! Some things never change!

Our beautiful daughter was born at 10:46pm. She was definitely ready to arrive in the world as she only took six pushes and she was out. It was the most beautiful thing I have ever done and would love to give birth again. My husband was able to deliver her (after the midwife caught her as she shot out) and placed her on my chest. It was a good couple of minutes before we even thought to see what sex she was. Our darling daughter, Brooke Daisy-James was born at 10:46pm to Led Zeppelin's 'Dazed and Confused' and could not have been more amazing!

One incredibly proud and happy Mummy!!

Chapter 28

Meet the Dads

Quite naturally, because this is a book about pregnancy, we have heard mostly from the Mums. After all, it is their body that experiences the changes, grows this little person and then evicts them after nine months.

However, having a baby is not just down to one person and whether Dad is part of the family group or separate from it, they are still a part of that child's life.

I wanted the Dads to have their say on parenthood: how they felt about becoming a parent and any advice they wanted to share.

So, here are their tales.

Name: Ben
Age: 32

Tell us about your relationship before getting pregnant. We were very close from the beginning, but after getting married and moving to the country we were as close as we'd ever been.

How did you feel about becoming a parent? I wasn't conscious of it straight away but once we were pregnant I was scared of two things – that I would love my child too much, and that they wouldn't love me at all.

Did you change any habits while your partner was pregnant? I've not exactly changed my habits – I can still be whiny, selfish, forgetful, useless or argumentative – but I have tried to be more aware of when I'm doing these things. Or, at least, to realise I've been a jerk and try to make up for it!

What worries you about being a Dad? That he'll get seriously hurt and I won't be able to help. That he'll do something he'll be ashamed of. That I'll disappoint him. That I'll let myself be grumpy or frustrated and take it out on him or my wife.

What are you looking forward to doing with your child? Talking with him about anything and everything. Answering his first question. Playing cricket in the garden. Telling him stories of my own. Introduce him as a big brother to his siblings.

How did you cope when your partner was in labour? Not very well at first! I struggled to stay awake and useful overnight, and had trouble empathising with her pain during the first hours. But I felt far more confident once the final labour began, and especially after she'd had the epidural. I tried to keep myself busy, with fetching water or keeping her cool but in the end I found that the best thing for me and for her was to keep talking, to keep physically close and in contact with her, and to keep asking how I could help.

How did you feel seeing (and holding) your child for the first time? Proud. Incredibly and over-whelmingly proud of my son for getting here, for being with us, for being alive and so wonderful.

Any top tips for other Dads-to-be? Trust your child, trust your partner, trust yourself. Don't let other people's experiences get in the way of your own experiences. Get as close as you can as often as you can for as long as you can.

ಐ ಐ ಐ ಛ ಛ ಛ

Name: Pete
Age: 33

Is this your first child? Yes.

Tell us about your relationship before getting pregnant. We've been together since 1997 and married since 2009. I always knew that I wanted to have children and we'd been trying for a couple of years.

How did you feel about becoming a parent? It was a bit of a shock, but only as much that when Lou was doing the pregnancy test we'd geared ourselves up to be disappointed! It was really exciting, and I couldn't wait to tell family about it!

Did you change any habits while your partner was pregnant? I certainly drank less during the pregnancy partly because Lou wasn't drinking, so we didn't really open a bottle of wine, etc. In terms of socialising with friends I don't think it had much of an impact at all!

We still managed to go on a couple of holidays – including a trip to Italy for a friend's wedding at 7 months! In hindsight maybe that holiday wasn't such a good idea as it was certainly more like hard work for Lou towards the end of it rather than relaxing.

What worries you about being a Dad? I just hope that I can be there for him whenever he needs me to be and just try to be a good dad to him in general.

What are you looking forward to doing with your child? Watching him grow up, first steps/words, playing music with him, holidays. Going for a beer with him (okay, that's a while off yet!).

How did you cope when your partner was in labour? Okay, I think…I was worried for Lou as I knew she wanted to try and stay clear of things like the heavy painkillers/assisted birth, and in the end she had both an epidural and forceps. However, the staff at the hospital were so good and I had every confidence in them.

How did you feel seeing (and holding) your child for the first time? It was pretty amazing. It's just so strange when they finally arrive! No amount of 'One Born Every Minute' can prepare you for it. He seemed so tiny and fragile, not sure that he was happy being out of his cosy home of nine months!

Any top tips for other Dads-to-be? Just be as supportive as you can of your partner and do whatever they ask of you. Also don't worry about life after the baby – you'll hear people telling you all sorts of scare stories about lack of sleep and how much your life is going to change, but once you hold your child in your arms, you'll realise that it just doesn't matter.

ও ও ও গ গ গ

Name: Stuart
Age: 38

Is this your first child? Yes.

Tell us about your relationship before getting pregnant. Amazing.

How did you feel about becoming a parent? Excited and nervous but I felt confident that Claire had experience with children and this made a lot of worries go away.

Did you change any habits while your partner was pregnant? Yes! I had fewer nights out as I felt guilty leaving her alone.

What worries you about being a Dad? I was just hoping that he would be healthy and not have any medical issues: this was my main worry.

What are you looking forward to doing with your child? Taking him to my business to show him around, family holidays, rough and tumble play.

How did you cope when your partner was in labour? I thought I did well, but panicked a bit at the beginning. She had issues afterwards so I was given Harry and I felt a rush of emotion. I got told off as the tea and toast was for her after labour but I thought the midwife had brought it for me!

How did you feel seeing (and holding) your child for the first time? Overwhelming emotions of love and responsibility.

ဆ ဆ ဆ ဆ ဆ ဆ

Name: Anthony
Age: 52

Is this your first child? No.

Tell us about your relationship before getting pregnant. Easy going, love, laughter and hanging out.

How did you feel about becoming a parent? Glad and happy.

Did you change any habits while your partner was pregnant? A little less socialising since I hung out with her the most.

What worries you about being a Dad? Not having enough energy.

What are you looking forward to doing with your child? Showing him how to be a real man, watching football and basketball games.

How did you cope when your partner was in labour? [I was] petrified when she had to undergo surgery.

How did you feel seeing (and holding) your child for the first time? That it was all worth it.

Any top tips for other Dads-to-be? Take it one day at a time.

ಐ ಐ ಐ ಐ ಐ ಐ

Name: Marcus
Age: 30

Is this your first child? Yes.

Tell us about your relationship before getting pregnant. A lot of holidays to America and boating in Norfolk on the spur of the moment. Pretty much impulsive weekend activities, very little forward planning.

How did you feel about becoming a parent? Tired, because I found out when I was half asleep! Later in the day I was ecstatic.

Did you change any habits while your partner was pregnant? I'm not much of a drinker and I still have NASCAR Sundays.

What worries you about being a Dad? When she becomes a teenager, potty training, being a responsible role model, sensible financial management, outgrowing our accommodation.

What are you looking forward to doing with your child? Teaching them stuff, toy shop shopping, Disneyland Florida, birthday parties, first Christmas.

How did you cope when your partner was in labour? There wasn't a lot I could really do. I was concerned for Beth as I couldn't make her feel better.

How did you feel seeing (and holding) your child for the first time? Conflicting emotions: elation for the baby and concern for the wellbeing of her mother.

Any top tips for other Dads-to-be? Remain calm – it's not as everyone makes it out to be!

ꜩ ꜩ ꜩ ꜩ ꜩ ꜩ

Name: Steve
Age: 34

Tell us about your relationship before getting pregnant. Laura and I had been together for five year, living together for two and had recently got married. Our lives apart from work involved dinner parties, holidays, weekend breaks, parties, cinema and basically enjoying life with ourselves, family and friends.

How did you feel about becoming a parent? Amazing. Our plan shortly after getting married was to start a family but I didn't have high expectations of getting pregnant so quickly – I thought at least we'd have a few months!

Did you change any habits while your partner was pregnant? Our habits and lifestyle have changed a lot but it doesn't feel like we're missing anything. We moved to a new city shortly after getting married/pregnant so we had a new routine in a new place and met lots of new people through NCT who were also expecting. As one door closes, many others have opened!

What worries you about being a Dad? Having more kids! How busy/hectic life will become as our daughter (and maybe her future brothers/sisters) grows up. The cost! How the relationship between

Laura and I will change with kids and finding time just for us.

What are you looking forward to doing with your child? Teaching her to ski! Christmas, Easter egg hunts, Halloween and Father's Day!

How did you cope when your partner was in labour? I think I did OK – I made sure I included Laura in the discussions so throughout we both felt we were in control on what happened to her. It helped to keep Laura calm and although we couldn't stick to the birth plan, afterwards and to this day we have no regrets about it.

How did you feel seeing (and holding) your child for the first time? After 42 hours of labour and no sleep I was pretty whacked but it was an incredible experience and almost too overwhelming to take in.

Any top tips for other Dads-to-be? Spend as much time as you can early on with your wife and baby, helping your wife to get used to doing as many things as you can before you go back to work, so she's comfortable getting out and about in foot, car, bus, train, etc, changing nappies and feeding not just at home but more importantly in cafes and shops. Then she'll be free to meet up with other new mums early on and vent all her worries and concerns about your baby and being mum in a like- minded group of people. She'll be happier and less stressed, which makes for a happy home (and baby!) to come to after work!

ဆ ဆ ဆ os os os

Name: Geoff
Age: 39

Is this your first child? Yes.

Tell us about your relationship before getting pregnant. It was very good but I believe my partner felt something was missing if we didn't have a child.

How did you feel about becoming a parent? Quite pleased but not dancing on the rooftops. A bit shocked that it happened so easily.

Did you change any habits while your partner was pregnant? No change when pregnant. Less TV watching since and no football games due to lack of money.

What worries you about being a Dad? That I will mess the child up and create a monster child, never-ending responsibility, lack of financial security.

What are you looking forward to doing with your child? Going to school functions and watching her perform in plays, etc, Christmas stuff like visiting Santa's grotto, having hugs, having a dance.

How did you cope when your partner was in labour? Distressed seeing her in pain but once I saw the pain relief work things were much calmer. Having a good midwife helped.

How did you feel seeing (and holding) your child for the first time? Very happy (not crying; emotional though, which surprised me) and I didn't want to give her over to her mother!

Any top tips for other Dads-to-be? Enjoy the freedom/flexibility while you can! Be prepared to waste lots of money on children's clothes that will either never be worn or worn only once. Be prepared to enjoy being covered in baby sick, spit or wee.

Be prepared to not want to put your child down and to want to cuddle her forever!

ဆ ဆ ဆ os os os

Some final thoughts and advice...

Rachel, a second-time Mum, offered some thoughts and advice which seemed to provide the perfect conclusion to this book. Here they are in full.

First: being a Mum is a noble task. But that noble task is made up of hundreds of menial tasks. The challenge is to not mistake menial for meaningless.

All the experts say that the early years are crucial, so every time you build a tower of blocks that is immediately knocked down, every time you clear up vomit or poo, or food thrown on the floor, every time it takes an hour to walk round the block because your toddler stops to look at every tiny spot on the pavement, every time you drag yourself out of bed in the middle of the night to see to a crying baby, every time you read their favourite book twenty times in one day, every time you do the third round of laundry and third bowl of washing up in one day, every time you are covered in paint or glue, every time you play hide and seek even though their 'hiding' place is always the same but you pretend not to know, every time you prioritise their needs over your own (which is pretty much all the time!), then you are building a foundation for the future.

Prioritise love and affection and fun and laughter over tidiness and order and efficiency. At the time it feels like total chaos and you long for more sleep, more order, more 'me time' ...but every older parent will tell you how quickly these early years go by and you never get them back.

(I am still learning these lessons every day! It's hard to keep a good perspective when you're in the thick of it!)

Second: get help!

Being a parent is the most rewarding but hardest job in the world and there will be days when you just cannot do it on your own. Don't be too proud to ask for help. Ask a friend or family member to do whatever it is that will help you feel better... Tidy your house, cook your dinner, take your baby out for a walk, be a shoulder to cry on, give you a massage, do your shopping, look after your baby while you go for a walk... Anything!

Don't be afraid to say you're not coping. Ongoing sleep deprivation can do crazy things to you and make you feel like you're going mad. Millions, if not billions of other people have been there too. They will sympathise and be only too glad to help.

Acronyms

There are lots of acronyms used in this book, mostly relating to conception and IVF procedures. To maintain the flow of the tales I didn't want to explain these in the text and so have decoded them here.

AF	Auntie Flo (your period)
AMH	Anti-mullerian hormone
AT	Actively trying
BB	Birth board (on BabyCentre)
BC	BabyCentre
BD	Baby dance (having sex)
BF	Breastfeeding
BFN	Big fat negative (on a pregnancy test)
BFP	Big fat positive (on a pregnancy test)
BMI	Body mass index
BP	Blood pressure
CBFM	Clear Blue Fertility Monitor
CD	Cycle day
CM	Cervical mucus
CPR	Cardiopulmonary resuscitation
CVS	Chorionic villus sampling
DH	Dear/darling husband
DPO	Days past ovulation
DTD	Doing the deed (having sex)
EC	Embryo collection
ECV	External cephalic version
EPO	Evening primrose oil
ET	Embryo transfer
EWCM	Egg white cervical mucus
FET	Frozen embryo transfer
FF	Formula feeding
FMU	First morning urine
FN	Fertility nurse
FS	Fertility specialist
GD	Gestational diabetes

HFEA	Human Fertilisation and Embryology Authority [UK]
IB	Implantation bleeding
ICSI	Intracytoplasmic sperm injection
IUI	Intrauterine insemination
IVF	In vitro fertilisation
LO	Little one
LOL	Laugh(ing) out loud
MC	Miscarriage
MIL	Mother-in-law
MW	Midwife
NCT	National Childbirth Trust
NHS	National Health Service
OH	Other half (partner)
OPK	Ovulation predictor kit
OV	Ovulation
PG	Pregnant
PMA	Positive mental attitude
PMT	Pre-menstrual tension
SA	Sperm/semen analysis
SCBU	Special care baby unit
SS	Symptom spotting
TBH	To be honest
TENS	Transcutaneous electrical nerve stimulation
TMI	Too much information
TTC	Trying to conceive

Glossary of terms

Many different terms are used in this book. The following list includes the ones I felt were most important.

Amniocentesis
A diagnostic test carried out during pregnancy. It can assess whether the unborn baby could develop, or has developed, an abnormality or serious health condition.

Anovulatory cycle
A menstrual cycle in which ovulation fails to occur.

Apgar scale
A simple, painless and effective test used by midwives and doctors to assess your new-born's health.

Braxton Hicks contractions
This is the muscles in your uterus tightening towards the end of your pregnancy. They are irregular and do not increase in intensity unlike labour contractions.

Clomid
The brand name for a medicine that blocks the effect of oestrogen in the body and is used in the treatment of infertility.

Cord prolapse
Where the umbilical cord slips through your cervix ahead of your baby. There's a danger the cord will be squashed during birth, cutting off your baby's oxygen supply.

Ectopic pregnancy
When a fertilised egg implants itself outside of the womb, usually in one of the fallopian tubes.

Egg sharing
An IVF treatment that brings together women who produce surplus eggs with those unable to produce eggs.

Endometriosis
A common condition in which small pieces of the womb lining (the endometrium) are found outside the womb.

Episiotomy
A cut in a woman's perineum which makes the opening of the vagina a bit wider, allowing the baby to come through it more easily.

Fibroids
Non-cancerous tumours that grow in or around the womb. The growths are made up of muscle and fibrous tissue and can vary in size.

Lap and dye test
A procedure where a coloured dye is injected into the fallopian tubes to check for blockages and other problems.

Microgynon
The brand name of a combined oral contraceptive pill.

Omeprazole
A medicine which is used in a number of conditions. One use is to treat stomach ulcers and to relieve heartburn and indigestion.

Ovitrelle
The brand name of a medicine which is used in female infertility. It may be used in women as part of an assisted reproductive technique such as IVF or in women who produce no eggs at all or too few eggs.

Polycystic ovaries
Contain a large number of harmless cysts that are no bigger than 8mm each. The cysts are under-developed follicles which contain eggs that haven't developed properly. Often these follicles are unable to release an egg, meaning ovulation doesn't take place.

Pre-eclampsia
A condition that affects some pregnant women usually during the second half of pregnancy (from around 20 weeks) or soon after their baby is delivered.

Propess
The brand name of a hormone pessary which works by relaxing the muscles of the cervix.

Prostaglandin
A hormone-like substance that causes your cervix to ripen, and which may stimulate contractions.

Sources:
www.nhs.co.uk, www.babycentre.co.uk,
www.babyhopes.com, www.eggsharing.com

Useful contacts

This is not intended to be comprehensive and all-embracing. Things move too fast to make such a list practical or useful and the Internet is better at dealing with that. Rather, it includes what I believe to be the more important organisations for those trying for, waiting for and then delivering a newborn.

Alphamom: American site with a good pregnancy calendar
www.alphamom.com

Breastfeeding help and support
www.kellymom.com
www.laleche.org.uk

Down's Syndrome: information and support
www.futureofdowns.com
www.downs-syndrome.org.uk

Forums, advice, etc.
www.babycentre.co.uk
www.netmums.com

HypnoBirthing: information
www.hypnobirthing.co.uk

IVF treatments: information
www.hfea.gov.uk (IVF)

The Miscarriage Association
www.miscarriageassociation.org.uk

National Childbirth Trust (NCT)
www.nct.org.uk

National Health Service (NHS)
www.nhs.co.uk

National Institute for Health and Clinical Excellence (NICE)
www.nice.org.uk

Post-natal depression: information and support
www.pni.org.uk

Index

A
acupuncture 9
adoption 82
afterbirth *see* placenta
alcohol 47–48, 57, 61, 69, 89, 106, 202
amniocentesis 69–71
anaemia 76, 100
anomaly scan see scans
antenatal classes (*see also* NCT) 79, 101, 129, 148
antibiotics 104
Apgar test 156, 191
assisted delivery
    forceps 111, 130, 134, 140, 141, 156, 177, 178, 203
    ventouse 134, 140, 142, 182, 192

B
BabyCentre 20, 21, 56, 75
birthing pools 130, 134, 155, 156, 169, 194–196
birth plans 84, 109, 128, 131–135, 207
bleeding 66, 91, 101, 107, 110, 119, 164, 185
    during sex 14
    first trimester 48, 51
    post-partum 79, 170
    spotting 52, 65, 107
blood blisters 79
blood pressure
    high 60, 118, 119, 133, 163, 164
    low 174
    test 22, 23, 166
blood tests 29, 36, 39–41, 53, 70
bowel movements 127, 129
    constipation 78, 98
    diarrhoea 16, 17
    during labour, 197
Braxton Hicks contractions 91, 101, 102, 109, 185, 195
breastfeeding 17, 94, 103, 112–114, 148, 149, 156, 171, 175, 184, 188, 192, 193, 199
breasts, sore 13, 16, 17, 37
breech babies 65, 109, 162, 197, 198
    and Caesarean section 45, 129, 162
    turning 65, 109, 129, 162, 163
bump 17–18, 36, 58, 71, 73, 74, 76, 95, 96, 100, 101, 108, 117–119, 152

C
Caesarean section
    elective 58, 67, 71, 129, 162, 163
    emergency 45, 66, 87, 111, 142, 159, 190, 197, 199
carpel tunnel 118

catheters 170, 171, 186
cervical sweep *see* induction of labour
cervix
    dilation 86, 87, 102, 110, 111, 140, 141, 155, 157, 160,
    164, 165, 169, 172, 174, 180, 182–184, 186, 189, 190,
    191–194, 196, 198
    'show' 109, 141, 155, 189
chorionic villus sampling (CVS) 68
cognitive behavioural therapy (CBT) 58
constipation *see* bowel movements
contraception
    coil 107
    condoms 59, 81, 83
    the pill 9, 41, 42, 58, 81, 98
contractions 86, 87, 102, 109–111, 134, 136–138, 140, 142,
145, 152, 155, 159, 160, 164, 165, 168, 169, 172–175, 178–
186, 189, 191–198
cravings 52, 61, 62, 78, 118

D
dating scan *see* scans
depression 25, 34, 106
    postnatal 104, 106
diabetes, gestational 65, 98, 119, 120, 134
Down's syndrome 67, 69–71,
drugs 106
    during pregnancy 90–94
    during labour *see* pain relief
    IVF drugs 24, 39–41
due date 50, 73, 85, 101, 109, 121, 157

E
ectopic pregnancy 9
egg sharing 35, 36
endometriosis 9, 20, 23, 26, 27
epidurals *see* pain relief
episiotomy111, 112, 178, 186, 192

F
fallopian tubes 9, 20, 22, 26, 27
feet, swollen 74, 117, 119
fertility clinic 18
fertility monitor 8
fertility test 18
fertility treatment 13
    ICSI 17, 36–39, 42–44
    IUI 8, 28–34
    IVF 9, 17, 28, 35, 37, 39, 40, 42, 149
fibroids 66, 76, 189
forceps delivery *see* assisted delivery
formula feeding 113

G

gas and air (entonox) *see* pain relief
glucose tolerance test (GTT) 74, 118

H

heartburn 74, 98, 118, 120
home birth 139, 155, 161
hormones 50, 90, 149
hospital bags 85, 120, 134, 143, 191
HypnoBirthing 129, 130, 133, 145, 184

I

incubator 167, 168
induction of labour 66, 85, 102, 131, 133, 139
    artificial rupture of membranes 66, 102, 110, 133, 141,
    155, 183, 186, 191
    cervical sweep 66, 102, 131, 155, 181, 183, 189
    pessary 85, 86, 157, 183
    prostaglandins 183
    Syntocinon drip (oxytocin) 133, 141, 183
in vitro fertilisation (IVF) *see* fertility treatment

J

jaundice 166, 167, 187

K

kidney infection 51, 64, 85

L

lap and dye *see* surgery
labour (birth stories) 154–199

M

maternity leave 55, 101, 152, 185
meconium 155, 156
membranes
    artificial rupture of 66, 102, 110, 133, 141, 155, 183, 186,
    191
    cervical sweep 66, 102, 131, 155, 181, 183, 189
    waters breaking 65, 91, 101, 137, 141, 142, 164, 168, 191,
    195
miscarriage 8–10, 17, 47, 48, 51, 53, 54, 59, 65, 69, 79, 83,
107, 108, 152
monitoring, foetal 64, 65, 86, 101, 110, 119, 156, 158, 164,
168, 179, 189, 192, 194
morning sickness 14, 41, 50–53, 56, 62, 73–75, 78, 85, 90, 96,
98, 100, 108, 115, 120
multiple pregnancy
    and IVF 45
    labour 197

N

National Childbirth Trust (NCT) 147, 193, 207
National Health Service (NHS) 7, 28, 31, 35, 67, 172

National Institute of Health and Clinical Excellence (NICE) 90
nausea 41, 52, 53, 61, 62, 73, 75, 91
neonatal unit (*see also* SCBU) 166

O
overdue babies 157

P
pain
    back pain 16, 85, 108, 152, 197
    headache 109
    hip and pelvic pain 74, 78, 98, 118
    stomach pain 16, 53, 107
pain relief
    diamorphine 177
    epidural 71, 86, 111, 130, 133, 134, 140, 142, 160–162,
    174, 175, 178, 184, 191, 192, 201, 203
    gas and air 86, 102, 133, 134, 138, 155, 158, 159, 162,
    165, 177, 181–183, 186, 192, 194, 196, 198
    paracetamol 27, 93, 136, 144, 155, 157, 168, 169, 178,
    181, 191
    pethidine 102, 111, 194
    spinal anaesthesia 156, 161
    TENS machine 134, 136, 144, 145, 152, 159, 162, 169,
    173, 177, 179, 181, 183, 193, 194
    water 102, 110, 169, 173
pelvic floor 78, 161
periods 7, 11, 12, 14, 16, 17, 25, 27, 35, 37, 38, 40–43, 50, 68
piles 78, 98
placenta 112, 161
    delivery of 103, 165, 187
    retained placenta 172
post-natal depression 104, 106
pre-eclampsia 118, 168
pregnancy test 7, 11–14, 52, 68, 81, 82, 89, 100, 202
premature babies 134, 141, 185, 187
prolapse cord 66

R
reflexology 15, 28, 34
relaxin 75

S
scans *see* ultrasound scans
sex 7, 14, 15, 22, 27, 31, 38, 90, 98
sex of baby 73, 114, 133
siblings 115
sickness (*see also* morning sickness)
    in labour 110, 111, 140, 156, 164, 192, 196–199
smoking 62, 90–93
special care baby unit (SCBU) 45, 71, 187, 188, 199
stitches 24, 103, 112, 170, 187
stretch marks 53, 79, 98, 101, 119
supplements 9, 21, 34, 35, 37, 100, 153

surgery (*see also* Caesarean section)
    lap and dye 20, 22, 23, 26
    post-partum 140, 161, 172
    pre-pregnancy 9, 149

T

TENS machine *see* pain relief
termination 82
tiredness 52–54, 73–76, 78, 79, 92, 95, 97, 100, 104, 108, 109, 117, 148, 149
tocophobia 58–60
transverse lie 45, 64, 197
trimesters
    first 48, 50–54, 61, 62, 65, 73, 78, 83, 151, 152
    second 50, 53, 70, 73–76, 83
    third 50, 85, 92, 117–121, 151, 152

U

ultrasound scans 30, 32, 35, 43, 53, 54, 65, 66, 69, 83, 107, 109, 114
    anomaly scan (20 weeks) 70, 73, 76
    dating scan (12 weeks) 46, 50, 73, 83
    Doppler 53
umbilical cord 56, 170
    around baby's neck 192
    cutting 161, 163, 184, 186, 192
    delayed cutting 130
    prolapse 66, 190
urine infection 52, 65, 74, 118
uterine hyper-stimulation 140, 152, 160

V

ventouse delivery *see* assisted delivery

W

waters breaking (naturally) 65, 91, 101, 137, 141, 142, 164, 168

Y

yoga 147, 152, 154